101 All-Time
Savoury Snacks

Elizabeth Jyothi Mathew

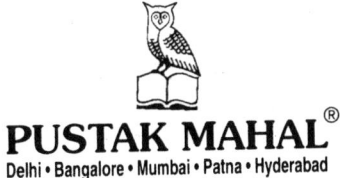

PUSTAK MAHAL®
Delhi • Bangalore • Mumbai • Patna • Hyderabad

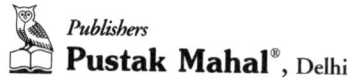

Publishers
Pustak Mahal®, Delhi

J-3/16, Daryaganj, New Delhi-110002
☎ 23276539, 23272783, 23272784 • *Fax:* 011-23260518
E-mail: info@pustakmahal.com • *Website:* www.pustakmahal.com

Sales Centre
10-B, Netaji Subhash Marg, Daryaganj, New Delhi-110002
☎ 23268292, 23268293, 23279900 • *Fax:* 011-23280567
E-mail: rapidexdelhi@indiatimes.com

Branch Offices
Bangalore: ☎ 22234025 • *Telefax:* 22240209
E-mail: pmblr@sancharnet.in • pustak@sancharnet.in
Mumbai: ☎ 22010941
E-mail: rapidex@bom5.vsnl.net.in
Patna: ☎ 3294193 • *Telefax:* 0612-2302719
E-mail: rapidexptn@rediffmail.com
Hyderabad: *Telefax:* 040-24737290
E-mail: pustakmahalhyd@yahoo.co.in

© **Pustak Mahal, Delhi**

ISBN 978-81-223-0667-5

Edition : 2009

The Copyright of this book, as well as all matter contained herein (including illustrations) rests with the Publishers. No person shall copy the name of the book, its title design, matter and illustrations in any form and in any language, totally or partially or in any distorted form. Anybody doing so shall face legal action and will be responsible for damages.

Printed at : Param Offsetters, Okhla, New Delhi-110020

Preface

In today's fast-paced world of globalisation and modernisation, the need for the modern woman to be able to cook for her family in the shortest possible time, has become not only a need but a necessity as well. Without any decrease in the quality of food, the modern woman wants to give her family the best in the least possible time.

This book is an attempt to help every housewife and mother to be able to provide those in between snacks at all times for her family. Instead of running out to the local bakery for snacks, this book is an attempt to encourage housewives to make all this at home. Not only will you be giving your family healthier food but your family will definitely enjoy the extra care and attention put in by you to prepare each of these recipes.

I hope that this book will be a delight not only to those who try out these recipes but also to those who eat the end-product as well. Remember that each time you open this book to cook, keep smiling. God bless you.

With warmest regards,
Elizabeth Jyothi Mathew

*Dedicated
to my Husband
Whom my Creator
has blest me with*

Contents

Basic Hints   9

1. **Vegetable Snacks**   11
   - Creamy Mushrooms on Toast   11
   - Mushroom Sandwich   12
   - Potato Scones   12
   - Health-Conscious Fries   13
   - Hot Fritters   14
   - Pineapple Sandwiches   14
   - Cheese Crispies   15
   - Easy Bread Patties   16
   - Easy Cheese Balls   16
   - Cheese Biscuits   17
   - Bread Rolls   17
   - Cheese Straws   18
   - Cheese Scones   19
   - Garlic Bread   19
   - Pumpkin Delight   20
   - Nut Delight   21
   - Italian Quick Snack   22
   - Baked Potato Cheese Delight   23
   - Chilli Cheese Puffs   23
   - Hot Garlic Bread   24
   - Little Party Sandwiches   24
   - Fried Potato Skins   25
   - Chips of a Different Kind   25
   - Hash Browns   26
   - Pappadum Cashew Delight   27
   - Yoghurt Dip with Crackers or Chips   28
   - Glazed Cheese Scones   29
   - Pinwheels   30
   - Onion Bhajias   31

	Baked Potatoes	32
	Bread Cups	33
	Cauliflower Cheese	34
	Golden Fritters	35
	Cheese Fritters	36
	Cheese Soufflé	37
	Corn Fritters	38
	Easy Damper	39
	Grilled Tomatoes	40
	Macaroni Cheese	41
	Onion Rings	41
	Spicy Potato Rounds	42
	Spicy Vegetable Fritters	43
	Quick Chilli Toast	44
	Rice Cakes	44
	Summer Tomatoes	45
	Yummy Potato Rounds	46
2.	**Egg Snacks**	**47**
	Stuffed Eggs	47
	Egg-White Cheese Balls	47
	Quick Sandwich	48
	Egg in Potato Nest	49
	Aberdeen Eggs	49
	Steamed Egg Snack	50
	Eggs Florentine	51
	Light Spanish Frittata	52
	Omelette Pizza	53
	Yummy Fluffy Omelettes	54
3.	**Seafood Snacks**	**55**
	Cold Prawn Balls	55
	Sardine Sandwich	55
	Bread Squares	56

Fish Loaf	56
Fish Sausage	57
Fish and Tomato Loaf	58
Crumbed Cheese Fish	58
Toasted Seafood Sandwich	59
Deep-Fried King Prawn	59
Chilli Prawn Croquettes	60
Butterfly Prawns	61
Pinwheel Sandwiches	61
Kofta Fish Balls	62
Crabmeat Balls	63
Fish Croquettes	64
Fish Pie	65
Fish Tempura	66
Prawn Cocktail	67
Prawn Pastry Puffs	68
4. Chicken Snacks	**69**
Cheese Canapes	69
Vegetable and Rice Custard	70
Almond Cream Dip	70
Chicken and Cucumber Double Decker	71
Grilled Chicken	71
Easy Chicken Wings	72
Chicken and Potato Scones	73
American Fried Chicken Wings	74
Crusty Rice Pizza	75
Chicken Cakes	76
Chicken Pastry	77
Crepe Delight	78
Chicken Rolls	79
Easy Gougere	80
Favourite Quiche	81
Savoury Pie	82

5. Meat Snacks		**83**
Beef Crescent Fry		83
Hamburgers		84
Meatballs and Cheese		85
Meat Tarts		86
6. Bacon Snacks		**87**
Horseback Snacks		87
Stuffed Pancakes		88
Instant Savoury Pie		89
Quick and Easy Pizza		89
Minced Meat Loaf		90
Fried Meat Cakes		91
Tips		**92**
Glossary		**93**

Basic Hints

Plan out your meals with a daily planner which plans ahead. Include one snack from this book everyday.

Read each recipe carefully.

Always get all Ingredients ready before actually starting your recipe. This will make cooking much easier.

Organize your kitchen so as to be able to produce as many 'goodies' as possible in the shortest possible time.

Remember to smile and enjoy your cooking. This makes the finished product even more tastier!

Above all, remember how blest we are to be able to cook and enjoy good food!

Abbreviations Used

tbsp	-	tablespoon
dsp	-	dessert spoon
tsp	-	teaspoon
lb	-	pound
oz	-	ounce
kg	-	kilogram
g	-	gram

1 dessert spoon is equivalent to 2 teaspoons.

Oven Temperatures

Electric	°C	°F
Slow	150	300
Moderate	180-200	375-400
Hot	240-250	475-500
Very hot	260	525-550

Weights and Measures

Use a 250 millilitre cup for measuring liquids. Have a set of 4 cups, measuring 1 cup, half cup, 1/3 cup and 1/4 cup.

Use a set of 4 spoons of accurate and equal measurements: tablespoon, teaspoon, half and quarter teaspoons.

Imperial	Metric
1/2 oz is replaced by	15 g
1 oz	30 g
2 oz	60 g
3 oz	90 g
4 oz (1/4 lb)	125 g
6 oz	185 g
8 oz (1/2 lb)	250 g
12 oz (3/4 lb)	375 g
16 oz (1 lb)	500 g
24 oz	750 g
32 oz (2 lb)	1000g (1 Kg)

Imperial	Metric cup	Metric (Liquid Measures)
2 oz	1/4 cup	30 ml
4 oz	1/2 cup	100 ml
5 oz	2/3 cup	150 ml
6 oz	3/4 cup	
8 oz	1 cup	250 ml

Vegetable Snacks

Creamy Mushrooms on Toast

Button mushrooms are ideal for this snack. Just make sure to have fresh cream on hand.

Ingredients *(Serves 4)*
- 8 slices of bread cut into diagonals
- 2 onions, sliced
- 2 cloves garlic, mashed
- 1 cup button mushrooms, sliced
- 4 tbsp butter
- 200 gms fresh cream
- Parsley or coriander leaves, chopped

Preparation
Heat a pan and add 2 tbsp of butter. Fry the bread pieces till golden. Remove and keep aside. In the same pan, add the remaining 2 tbsp of butter and sauté onions and garlic for about 3 minutes. Add the mushrooms and cook for another 5 minutes. Add the cream, salt and pepper. Remove from flame and pile this mixture onto each slice of bread. Serve garnished with the leaves.

Mushroom Sandwich

Try this triple sandwich full of goodness and nutrition instead of the usual rice and curry and watch inches disappear!!

Ingredients *(Serves 4)*

- 8 slices of bread
- 1 tsp butter
- 1 cup button mushrooms, sliced
- 1/2 cucumber sliced
- 1/2 cup paneer cubes, cooked in oil and drained
- 2 tsp chopped mint
- 1/2 orange, skinned and cut into thin slices

Preparation

In 1 tsp of butter, saute the mushrooms till cooked. Season with salt and lots of pepper. Layer each slice of bread with cucumber, then orange, paneer and finally with mushrooms. Cover with another slice of bread and garnish with mint leaves. Serve cut into diagonals and enjoy.

Potato Scones

What better idea than to make scones out of ordinary potatoes. Just be sure to serve them hot.

Ingredients *(Serves 8)*

- 1 kg boiled potatoes, cooled
- 2 tbsp butter
- Salt and pepper to taste
- 3 oz plain flour (or more as desired)
- 2 tsp of butter (or more as required)

Preparation

Mash potatoes and mix with the butter and salt. Work in as much flour as needed to roll out the mixture. Cut into rounds with a cutter and prick each scone with a fork. Heat a pan and put in 2 tsp of butter. Cook scones in this greased pan for about 3 minutes on each side. Serve hot with extra butter and eat hot.

Health-Conscious Fries

Terrified of French fries because of all that oil? Try these health-conscious fries which are not only guilt-free but oil-free as well.

Ingredients (Serves 6)

- 1 kg potatoes, washed and peeled
- 2 egg-whites, beaten
- Salt and pepper to taste
- 1/2 tsp chilli powder

Preparation

Slice the potatoes horizontally. Cut into the size of thick matchsticks. In a bowl, mix all the ingredients together, making sure that each potato piece is coated with the egg-white mixture. Place in a single layer in a baking dish and bake till golden brown. Serve hot with tomato sauce.

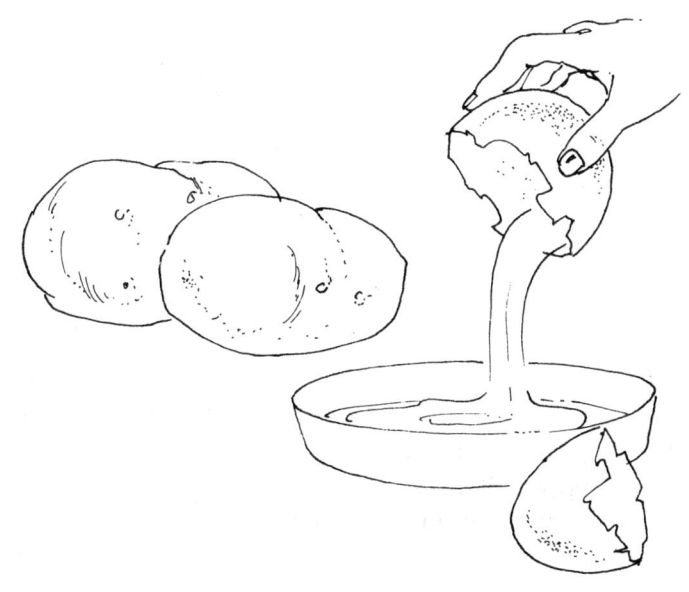

Hot Fritters

Simple easy-to-make fritters are always welcome in any home. The next snack is no exception.

Ingredients *(Serves 2)*

- 4 tbsp flour, sifted
- 2 tbsp chopped onion
- 1 clove garlic, smashed
- 1 egg, beaten
- Milk to make 1 cup of liquid with egg
- 1/2 cup grated cheese
- 1 tsp baking powder
- Oil for deep-frying

Preparation

Mix the flour, salt and pepper in a bowl. Add the onion, and garlic. Mix and add the egg and milk. Beat to form a batter. Then mix in the cheese and baking powder. Drop teaspoonfuls into hot oil. Fry till golden brown.

Pineapple Sandwiches

How about some pineapple sandwiches for a change? A fruity flavour in a savoury dish.

Ingredients *(Serves 2)*

- 1 cup, cheese spread
- 1/4 cup almonds, toasted and chopped
- 1/2 cup pineapple, chopped
- Salt and pepper to taste

Preparation

Drain the chopped pineapple thoroughly in a sieve. Add the pineapple to the cheese in a bowl. Add the almonds, salt and pepper. Blend well. Spread filling onto slices of soft bread and serve cut into diagonals.

Cheese Crispies

An ideal snack for children, the next recipe is sure to keep your children busy for some time.

Ingredients *(Serves 4)*

- 240 g butter
- 180 g cheese, grated
- 1/4 kg flour, sifted with 2 tsps of baking powder
- 2 cups cornflakes, crushed
- 1 egg and 1 egg-yolk, beaten together with 1 tbsp milk
- Salt and pepper to taste

Preparation

Cream butter well and add the rest of the ingredients. Mix well. Take small portions of the dough and roll out between 2 sheets of plastic wrap. Cut into different shapes with cookie-cutters and place on greased baking sheets. Bake for about 15 minutes till golden. Serve and watch it disappear before your very eyes.

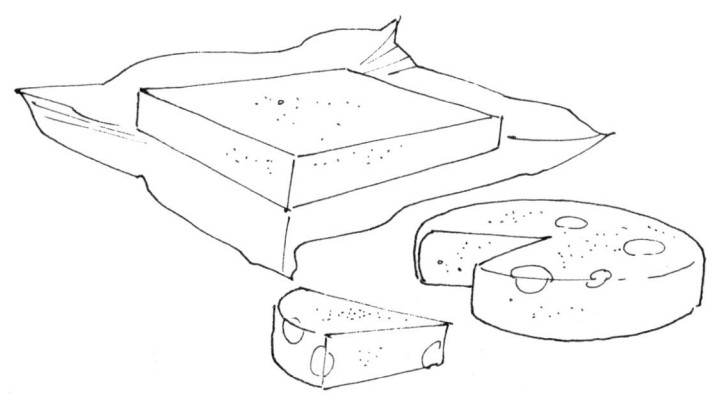

Easy Bread Patties

This is probably one of the easiest recipes you have ever tried out. With the simplest of ingredients, a nutritious snack is on the table!

Ingredients *(Serves 6)*

- 4 slices of bread, soaked in a little milk
- 1/2 kg potatoes, boiled and mashed
- 2 onions, chopped finely
- 1 tbsp spring onions, chopped
- 1 egg, beaten
- Salt and pepper to taste

Preparation

Mash the bread and add to the potatoes. Mix well. Add the rest of the ingredients and mix till it becomes one big lump. Moisten hands with water and make into little patties of any desired shape and deep-fry in hot oil. Serve hot with sliced onions and tomato sauce.

Easy Cheese Balls

This is an easy way to make cheese balls. Double the quantity and you have a snack enough for a large party.

Ingredients *(Serves 2)*

- 100 g flour, sifted with 1 tsp baking powder
- 50 g cheese, grated
- 25 g butter
- 1 egg, beaten
- Milk to mix
- Oil for deep-frying

Preparation

In a bowl, rub in the butter into the sifted flour till the mixture is crumbly. Add half the grated cheese and the egg. Mix in milk as required to make a fairly stiff dough. Shape the dough into small balls and deep-fry till golden brown. Serve hot garnished with the remaining grated cheese.

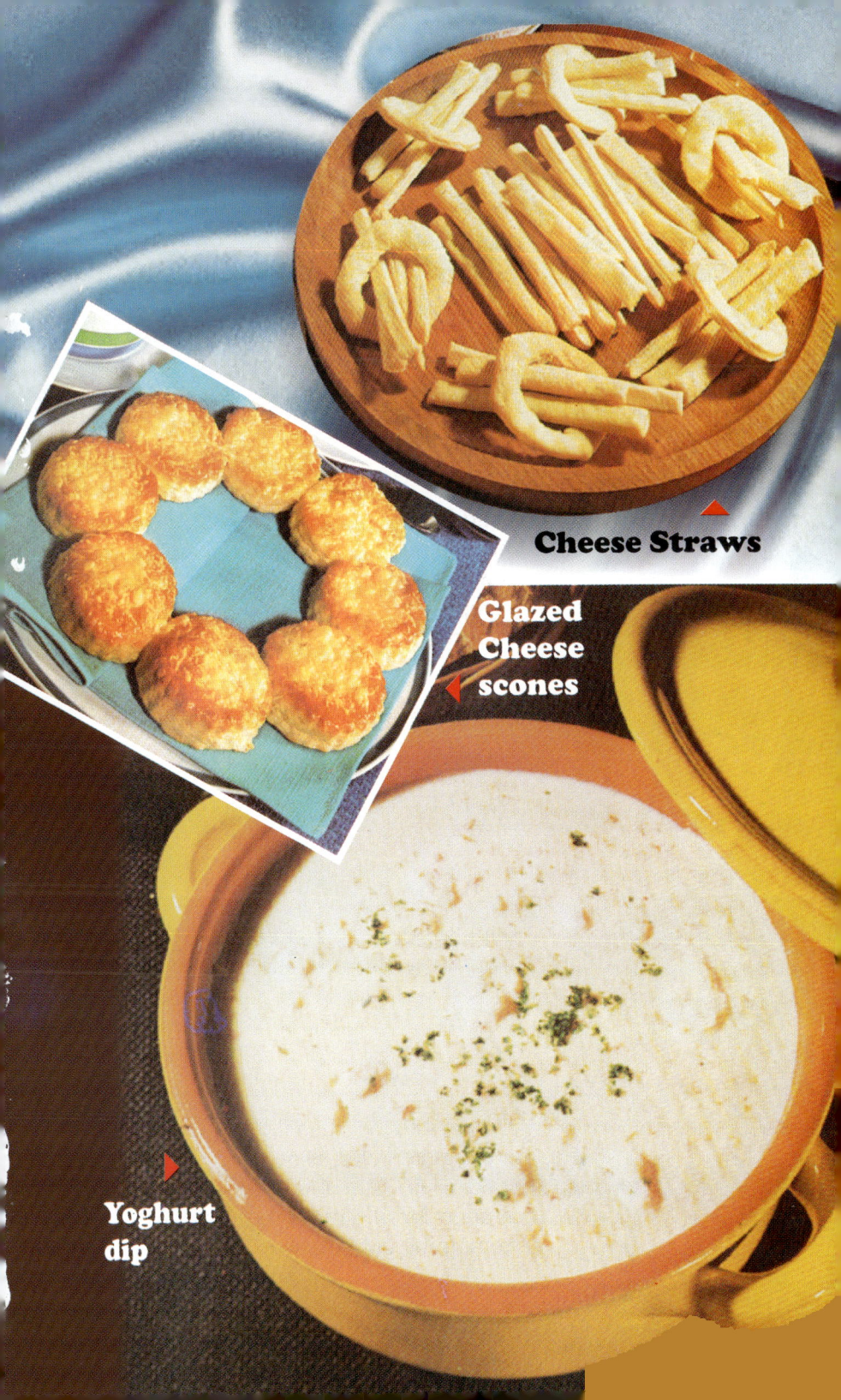

Cheese Straws

Glazed Cheese scones

Yoghurt dip

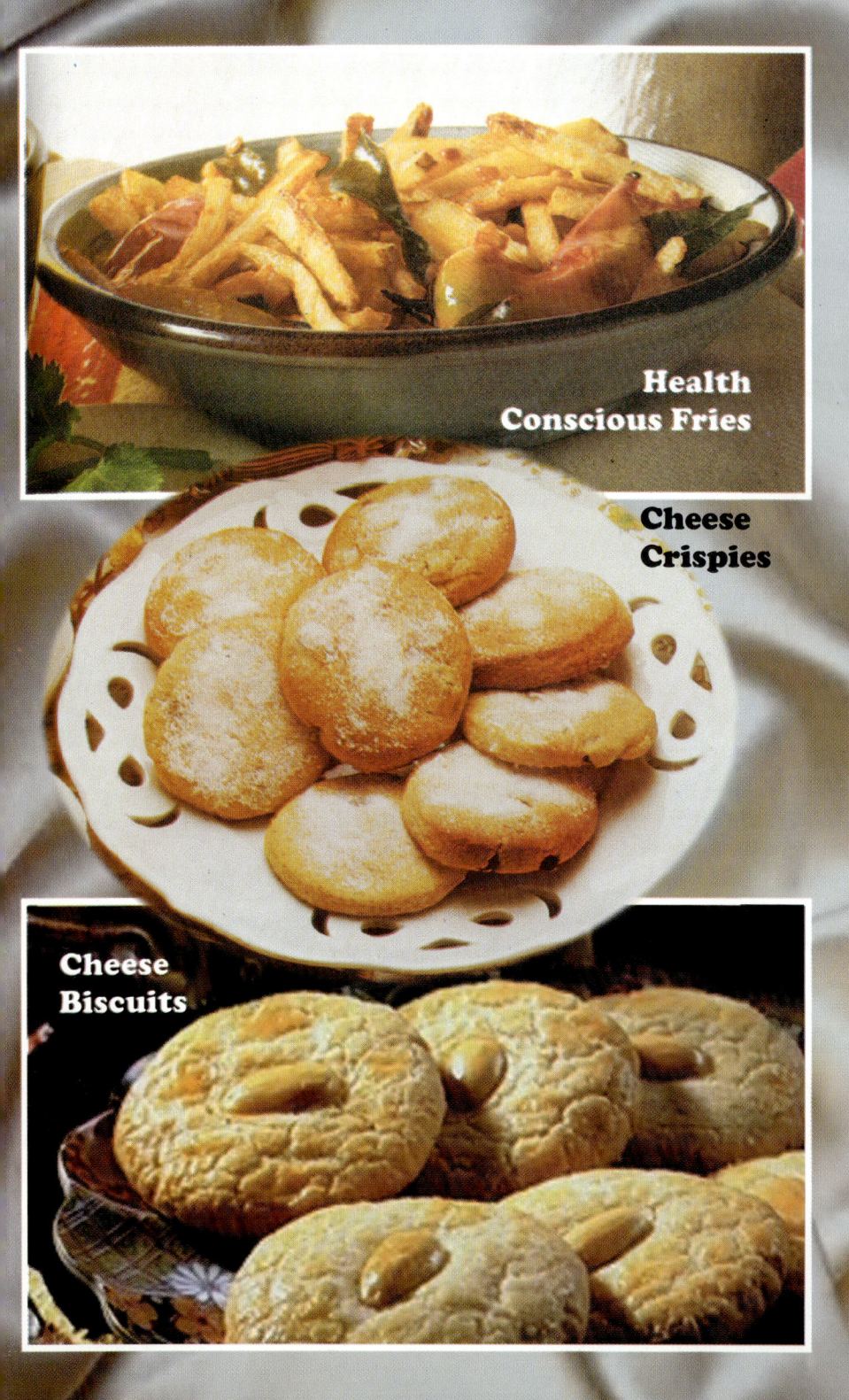

Cheese Biscuits

Biscuits with a difference, the next snack cuts calories because it is baked.

Ingredients (Serves 4)
- 75 g plain flour
- 25 g butter
- 50 g cheese, grated
- Milk to mix

Preparation
Sift the flour into a bowl and rub in the butter until the mixture resembles breadcrumbs. Add half the cheese and milk to form a stiff dough. Knead the dough lightly on a floured board and roll out. Cut into fancy shapes and brush with milk. Sprinkle the remaining cheese on each biscuit and put on a greased baking tray. Bake for about 15 minutes till golden brown. Serve garnished with extra grated cheese.

Bread Rolls

Try these little bread rolls which will keep your guests fascinated!

Ingredients (Serves 2)
- 5 slices of bread, crusts removed
- 3 tbsp butter
- 2 tsp of chopped coriander leaves
- 2 tbsp mushrooms, chopped and fried in butter
- 1 tsp lemon juice
- 1 boiled egg, chopped

Preparation
Flatten each slice of bread with a rolling pin. Mix the rest of the ingredients together in a small bowl. Put some of this filling lengthwise in each slice of bread. Roll up each slice of bread tightly and cover with foil. Chill till serving time.

Cheese Straws

These are straws of a different kind.

Ingredients *(Serves 4)*

- 1 1/2 cups (150g) plain flour
- 100 g butter, melted
- 2 tbsp grated cheese
- 1 egg-yolk
- Ice water
- Salt and pepper to taste
- Pinch of turmeric powder

Preparation

Sift the flour, salt , pepper and turmeric. Rub in the butter till the mixture resembles breadcrumbs. Stir in the cheese, egg-yolk and enough ice water to hold the dough together. Roll out to about 6mm (1/4 inch) thick and slice into straws, 10cm long and 6mm wide. Arrange them a little apart from each other on greased baking trays and bake for about 7 minutes till crisp and golden. Serve warm.

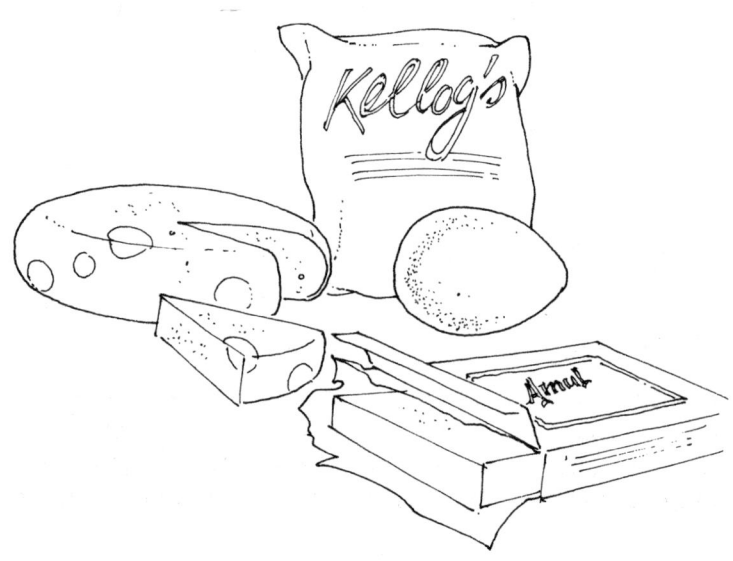

Cheese Scones

Get your pastry board ready to roll out some scones which are baked to perfection.

Ingredients *(Serves 2)*

- 100 g flour, sifted with 2 tsp baking powder
- 50 g butter
- 50 g cheese, grated
- Salt to taste
- Milk to mix

Preparation

In a bowl, rub in the butter into the sifted flour till the mixture resembles breadcrumbs. Add the cheese and milk to form a stiff dough. Knead lightly. Roll out the pastry until 2 cms thick on a floured board and cut into rounds. Arrange on a greased baking tray and brush with milk. Bake for about 15 minutes in a moderate oven. Serve hot with extra butter.

Garlic Bread

Not only is this an easy favourite but filling as well.

Ingredients *(Serves 4)*

- 8 slices of bread
- 60 g butter
- 1 tbsp garlic, crushed

Preparation

Preheat oven. Melt the butter on a low heat. Mix in the crushed garlic and brush on each slice of bread. Cut each slice either into diagonals or into 3 rectangles. Place the bread pieces, butter side up on to a baking sheet and bake for about 30 mins till golden brown. Serve hot with soup.

Pumpkin Delight

A snack with a difference. Ideal for the vegetarians and the health buffs.

Ingredients *(Serves 4)*

- 3/4 kg pumpkin, cut into 1$\frac{1}{2}$ inches thick pieces
- 60 g butter
- 2 tbsp golden syrup
- 3/4 cup breadcrumbs
- Salt and pepper to taste

Preparation

Preheat the oven. Trim off the skin of the pumpkin and arrange in a greased shallow baking dish. Season with salt and pepper. Cover and bake for about 1/2 an hour. Meanwhile melt butter and the golden syrup in a pan over low heat. Stir in the breadcrumbs and pour it over the baked pumpkin. Bake uncovered for another 15 to 20 minutes and serve.

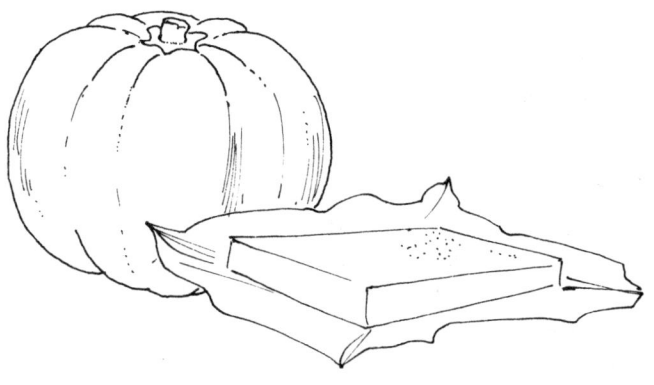

Nut Delight

This snack is sure to be finger licking good. Warning—you might not stop eating!

Ingredients *(Serves 4)*

- 1/4 kg of mixed nuts, (eg. almonds, cashews, peanuts etc.)
- 1 tbsp oil
- 1 tbsp butter
- 1 clove garlic, crushed
- Rock salt
- 1/2 tsp chilli powder

Preparation

Blanch the almonds in hot water and remove the skin. Or else toast for a couple of the minutes and rub off the skins. Heat the oil and butter in a frying pan and fry the garlic till there is an aroma. Add the nuts and reduce the heat. Fry till crisp and golden for about 5 minutes. Drain on paper towels and toss in the rock salt and chilli powder. Serve hot.

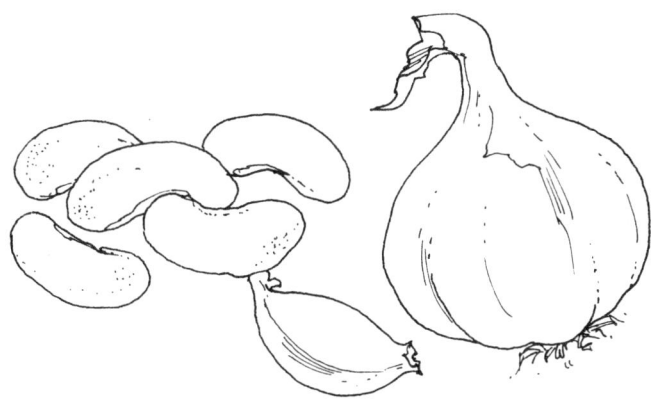

Italian Quick Snack

A simple bread based yummy snack ideal for vegetarians....

Ingredients *(Serves 6)*

- 12 slices of bread, cut into circles
- 100 g butter
- 2 tbsp plain flour
- 1 cup milk
- 1/4 cup grated cheese
- 1 cup mushrooms, chopped finely
- 2 tbsp grated cheese, extra
- Salt and pepper to taste
- Strips of capsicum for decoration

Preparation

Cut either 2 circles or one single circle from each slice of bread. Melt 40g of the butter and brush the bread circles with the butter. Place on the oven tray and bake for 10 minutes till golden brown. Melt extra butter in a pan and add the flour. Cook for a minute and add the milk. Stir till the mixture boils and thickens. Remove from heat and add the cheese, salt and pepper. Mix well. Spread this mixture evenly over each bread circle and sprinkle the extra cheese. Decorate with the capsicum strips . Bake in a hot oven for 5 minutes and serve.

Baked Potato Cheese Delight

Transform simple potato and cheese to a baked delight.

Ingredients *(Serves 6)*

- 1/2 cup boiled potato, mashed
- 3/4 cup (3 oz) plain flour, sifted
- 1/4 cup (2 oz) butter
- 1 egg, beaten
- 6 tbsp cheese, grated
- Extra cheese, grated

Preparation

Rub butter into the flour. Add the salt and pepper. Add the cheese and mashed potato which should be cold. Roll out to 1/8 inch thickness on a floured board and cut into shapes. Brush each with egg and sprinkle with cheese. Bake in a moderate oven for about 20 minutes. Store in an airtight tin, provided you have leftovers.

Chilli Cheese Puffs

Try this light snack and see how simple eggs-whites can be turned into a culinary delight.

Ingredients *(Serves 4)*

- 2 egg-whites, beaten stiffly
- 1/4 cup grated cheese
- 1/2 tsp chilli powder
- Salt and pepper to taste
- Oil for deep frying
- Extra grated cheese

Preparation

Beat egg-whites till stiff. Then add the cheese and the seasonings. Heat the oil in a pan and drop in small teaspoons of the mixture and fry until golden brown. Drain. Just before serving sprinkle with the extra grated cheese.

Hot Garlic Bread

Hot garlic bread is a welcome to any guest. Served with soup, salad or by itself, garlic bread is quite a sensation.

Ingredients *(Serves 8)*
- 1 loaf of bread
- 1/2 cup butter, melted
- 2 cloves garlic, crushed
- Salt

Preparation

Cream butter and garlic together. Slash the bread diagonally into 3/4 inch slices without going through right to the bottom. Spread the garlic butter generously between the slices. Wrap loaf in foil and heat in a hot oven for about 20 minutes. Serve hot.

Little Party Sandwiches

How about using the pastry cutter for something entirely different.... making sandwiches?

Ingredients *(Serves 6)*

- 1/2 loaf sliced bread
- 6 slices of cheese
- Salt and pepper to taste
- Butter or ghee to fry

For Batter
- 1 egg, beaten
- 1 tbsp flour
- 2 tbsp milk

Preparation

With a small pastry cutter, cut the cheese and bread into circles. Butter the bread and sprinkle with salt and pepper. Cover half the rounds with cheese. Press the other rounds firmly on top, making sandwiches. Dip these sandwiches into the batter and fry in the butter or ghee till golden brown. Drain and serve garnished with a little grated cheese.

Fried Potato Skins

We've all tried French fries, but what about the next dish? Next time you throw away potato skins, think of all that potential snack food going to waste.

Ingredients *(Serves 6)*

- 6 potatoes
- Oil for deep-frying

Preparation

Prick potatoes all over with a fork and bake in a pre-heated oven for about 1 hour or until cooked. Cool. Cut the potatoes in half and scoop out the flesh leaving a shell of 6 mm. Use the centres for another dish. Slice each skin into 4 pieces and deep-fry in hot oil till brown and crisp. Serve with mayonnaise.

Chips of a Different Kind

Try these chips for a change. Let me assure you it is of a different kind.

Ingredients *(Serves 5)*

- 1/2 kg white sweet potato, sliced thinly
- Oil for deep-frying

For Mayonnaise

- 1/2 cup mayonnaise
- 1 tbsp coriander leaves, chopped
- 2 tbsp yoghurt
- 1/2 tsp chilli powder

Preparation

Heat oil and deep-fry the slices of sweet potato until lightly browned and crisp. Drain on absorbent paper and serve with the mayonnaise.

For the mayonnaise: Mix all the ingredients together well and serve in a nice bowl. Enjoy.

Hash Browns

A favourite with Americans, it will be no surprise if this dish becomes our favourite too!

Ingredients *(Serves 2)*
- 4 potatoes, grated
- 2 bacon rashers, chopped
- 1/3 cup oil
- 2 tbsp butter
- 2 cloves garlic, chopped
- 1/4 kg mushrooms, chopped roughly
- 2 tomatoes, sliced

Preparation

Mix the potatoes and bacon in a bowl. Heat oil and drop about 2 tbsp of potato mixture in the oil and flatten into a round shape. Cook till brown on both sides and drain on absorbent paper. Repeat with the rest of the potato mixture. Heat butter and fry the garlic and mushrooms till cooked. Remove. Fry tomatoes on both sides and drain. Serve the mushroom mixture and the tomatoes along with the hash browns.

Pappadum Cashew Delight

What do you do with extra pappadums in the house? Make a snack of course!

Ingredients *(Serves 6)*

- 6 pappadums, quartered and deep-fried
- 1 tbsp oil
- 1/4 cup curry leaves
- 2 medium onions, finely chopped
- 2 tbsp celery, chopped
- 2 tbsp capsicum, finely chopped
- 1/4 kg mushrooms, sliced
- 8 eggs, lightly beaten
- 1/4 cup spring onion, minced

Preparation

Heat the oil. Add the curry leaves till crisp. Then add the next four ingredients and cook till the onions turn soft. Pour the eggs to cover the ingredients in the pan. Cook till the eggs are cooked. Cut the omelette into thick strips and serve mixed with the pappadums, spring onions and spiced cashews.

To make Spiced Cashews: Heat 1 tsp oil in a pan and add 1 cup of raw cashews. Cook till light brown. Add 1 teaspoon chilli powder, 1/2 tsp coriander powder, 1/2 tsp ground cumin, salt and pepper. Mix and cook till fragrant for a little more than a minute.

Yoghurt Dip with Crackers or Chips

Try this for a children's party and see the dip finish right before your very eyes!!

Ingredients (Serves 8)

- 280 ml thick yoghurt
- 1/4 cup spring onions, chopped
- 1/2 cup cucumber, chopped
- Few drops tabasco sauce
- Few drops Worcestershire sauce
- Few drops lemon juice
- Salt and pepper to taste

Preparation

Place the yoghurt in a large mixing bowl. Add the spring onions, cucumber, lemon juice, the sauces, salt and pepper. Mix and serve in a decorative bowl with crackers or potato chips.

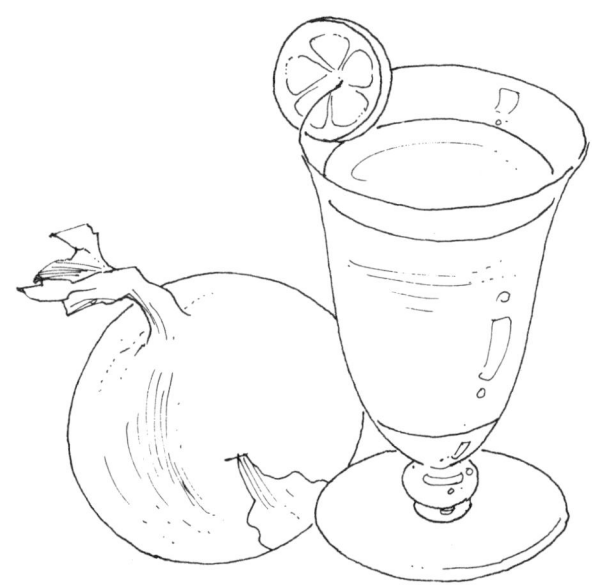

Glazed Cheese Scones

Always have cheese on hand to make quick snacks like the this one.

Ingredients *(Serves 4)*

- 240 g flour, sifted with 2 tsp baking powder
- 1 onion, chopped
- 60 g cheese, grated
- 45 g butter, melted
- 3/4 cup milk
- Salt and pepper to taste

For the glaze
- Beat together 1 egg and 1 tsp milk

Preparation

In a bowl mix the sifted flour, onion, cheese, salt and pepper together. Add the butter to the milk and pour into the dry ingredients. Mix to a soft dough with a spoon. Turn out onto a lightly floured board and roll out dough to about 2 cms thick between 2 sheets of plastic wrap. Cut into circles or any desired shape. Place on lightly greased baking trays and bake for about 20 minutes till golden. Brush scones immediately with the egg glaze.

Pinwheels

These pinwheels are a treat especially for little kids who like wheels.

Ingredients *(Serves 2)*

- 100 g flour
- 2 level teaspoons baking powder
- 50 g butter
- 50 g cheese, grated
- Milk to mix
- 50 g grated cheese, extra
- Salt to taste

Preparation

Sift the flour, baking powder and salt into a bowl. Rub in the butter coarsely. Add the cheese and milk to form a stiff dough. Knead lightly on a floured board. Roll out dough into a rectangle 1 cm thick. Brush with melted butter or milk. Sprinkle with the extra grated cheese and roll up tightly. Cut into slices 2 cms thick and arrange on a greased baking tray. Bake for 15-20 minutes in a moderate oven till light brown. Serve garnished with grated cheese.

Onion Bhajias

Plain ol' onions can be turned into a delightful snack.

Ingredients *(Serves 4)*
- 2 tbsp oil
- 1/2 tsp mustard seed, ground
- 1 tsp fenugreek seed, ground
- 1 tsp turmeric powder
- Pinch of chilli powder
- Salt to taste
- 1 egg
- 1 cup gram flour
- Oil for deep-frying
- 2 onions, big, chopped fine

Preparation
Heat the oil and fry the ground spices for a minute. Add the onion and stir till well-mixed. Turn down the heat, cover, and cook till the onion is tender but not mushy. Leave the mixture to cool. Add in the gram flour, salt and egg. Stir well. Fry 1 tsp of the mixture in hot oil turning them almost immediately. As soon as they become puffy and golden brown, remove and drain on paper towels. Serve warm.

Baked Potatoes

Who would have thought that ordinary potatoes could be turned into a culinary delight!

Ingredients *(Serves 4)*
- 8 large potatoes, washed and wiped
- Melted butter
- Salt and pepper to taste
- 1 cup chopped cucumber
- 1 cup cooked mushrooms, sliced
- 2 large tomatoes, skinned and chopped
- Coriander leaves or parsley, chopped
- 8 rashers of bacon, fried and rolled

Preparation

Prick the potatoes with a fork to prevent the skin from bursting. Brush with melted butter all over. Place on a baking tray and bake in a moderately hot oven for about 1- $1^1/_2$ hours. After cooking the potatoes, make a cross at the top of each potato. Scoop out the pulp gently taking care not to tear the skin of the potato. Mash the pulp and season with salt and pepper. To it add, cucumber, mushrooms, tomatoes and parsley. Fill each of the 8 potato jackets with this mixture. Top each with a bacon roll and bake for another 5 minutes. Serve hot.

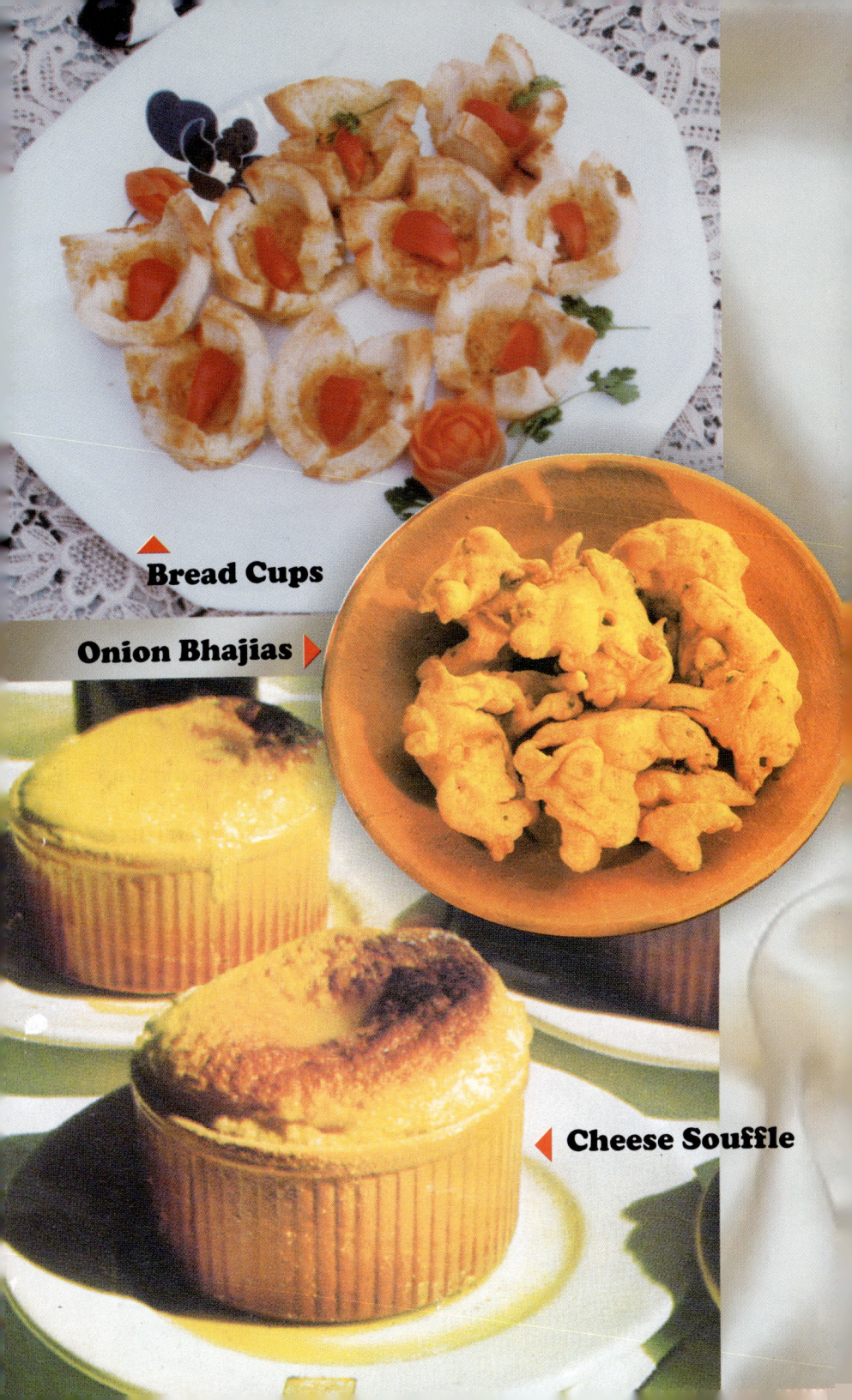

Bread Cups

Onion Bhajias

Cheese Souffle

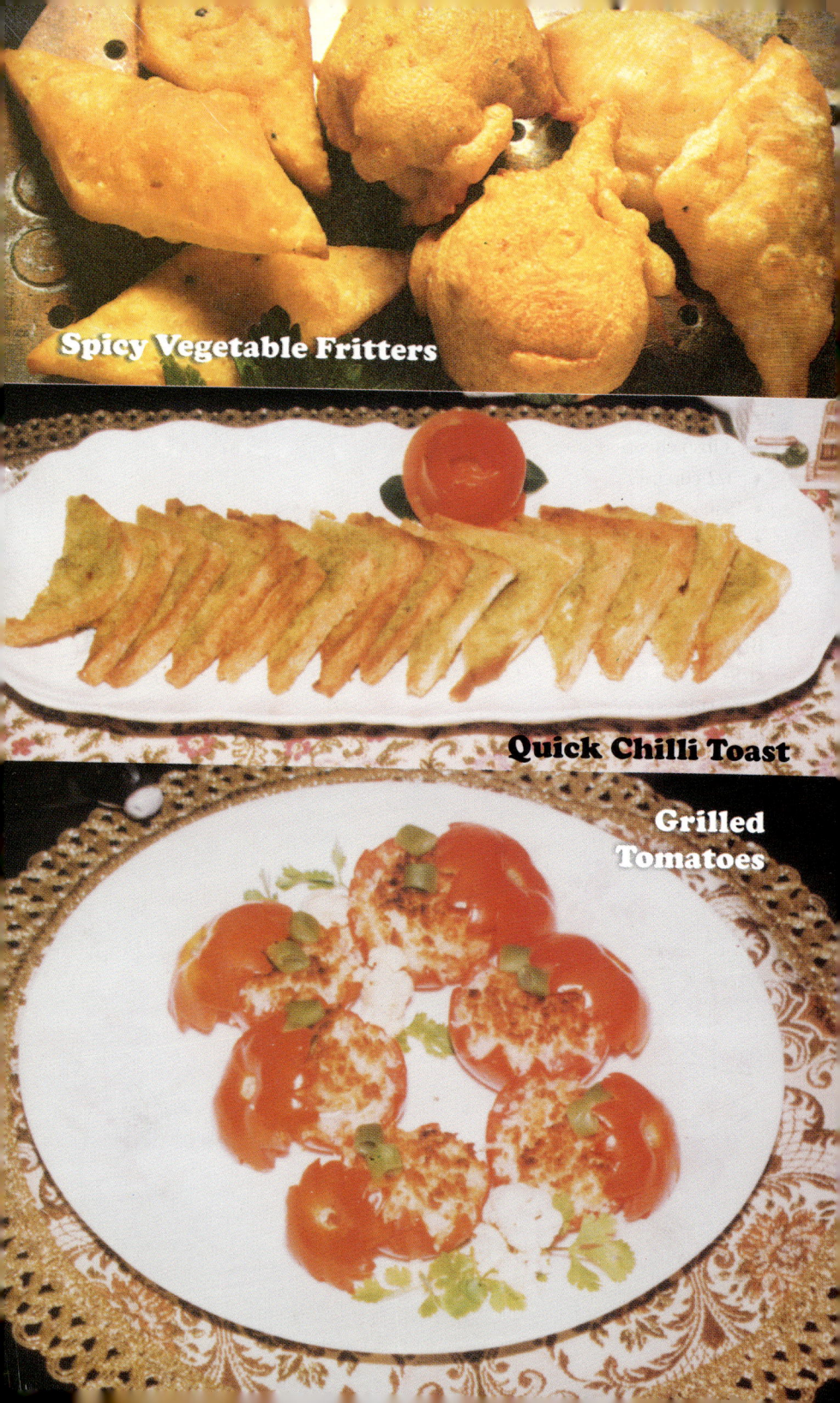

Bread Cups

Instead of serving bread in the usual way, try these bread cups for a change.

Ingredients *(Serves 4)*

- 8 slices bread, crusts removed
- 2 oz butter
- 2 eggs
- 4 oz paneer, crumbled
- 3 tbsp cheese, grated
- 1/2 cup milk
- Salt and pepper to taste
- 2 tomatoes, cut into quarters

Preparation

Butter each slice of bread and place each bread buttered side down into patty tins or baking cups. Whisk eggs along with paneer, cheese, milk and seasoning. Divide this mixture equally into each bread cup and bake in a moderate oven for about 20 minutes. Serve hot garnished with the tomato quarters.

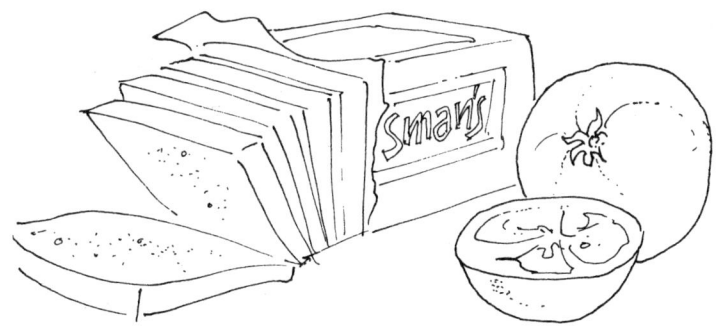

Cauliflower Cheese

Cauliflower has not tasted so good. Try it and you'll know exactly what I mean.

Ingredients *(Serves 4)*

- 1 medium size cauliflower
- 3 tbsp crisp breadcrumbs
- 1/2 cup, cheese, grated
- 2 oz grated cheese
- Cheese sauce (recipe below)

Preparation

Soak cauliflower in cold water for about 15 minutes. After separating it into florets, cook covered in boiling salted water. Arrange in buttered ovenproof dish. Pour the cheese sauce over. Cover with breadcrumbs and then grated cheese. Bake in a hot oven (425° F) until browned on top. Serve hot.

To make cheese sauce: In a pan, heat 2 tbsp butter. Add one chopped onion. Cook for 2 minutes and add 1 tbsp flour. Quickly add 1/2 litre milk and the cauliflower stock. Keep stirring till the mixture thickens.

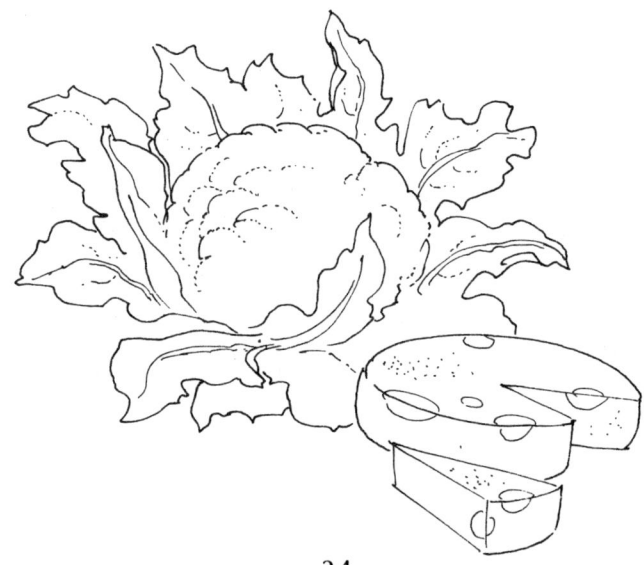

Golden Fritters

How about golden fritters for a real treat? Golden fritters are made of nothing but ordinary cauliflower.

Ingredients *(Serves 6)*

- 1 cauliflower, cut into florets
- 1/2 cup besan
- 1/4 cup self-raising flour
- 1/4 tsp bicarbonate of soda
- 2 cups water
- 1 egg
- 3/4 cup plain yoghurt
- 1/2 tsp ground cumin

Preparation

Wash the cauliflower. Dry it well. Combine the besan, flour, cummin and the soda in a bowl. Make a well in the centre. Beat the water, egg and yoghurt. Using a wooden spoon, mix this into the dry ingredients. Stir until smooth and free of lumps. Keep aside for 10 minutes. Heat oil for deep-frying. Dip the florets into the batter and lower into the oil. Cook until golden. Drain on paper towels. Serve hot.

Cheese Fritters

This mixture can be prepared 3 hours before needed and kept covered. Fry as required. A favourite with kids.

Ingredients *(Serves 6)*

- 80 g butter
- 1 cup water
- 1 cup plain flour
- 3 eggs, lightly beaten
- 1/2 cup grated cheese
- Salt and pepper to taste
- Oil for deep-frying

Preparation

Put water and butter in a pan and bring to the boil. When the water starts boiling, add the flour, salt and pepper all at once. Stir vigorously until the mixture leaves the sides of the pan. Add the beaten eggs, a little at a time beating well after each addition. Stir in the cheese. Heat some oil in a frying pan and drop in rounded teaspoons of mixture. Fry until lightly browned and cooked through. Repeat with the rest of the mixture. Drain on kitchen paper and sprinkle with a little extra grated cheese. Serve hot.

Cheese Soufflé

For those of you who like cheese, this will definitely be a favourite.

Ingredients *(Serves 2)*

- 5 tbsp butter
- 5 tbsp flour
- 1½ cups milk
- Salt to taste
- 6 eggs, separated
- 1 cup cheese

Preparation

In a saucepan, melt the butter and add flour, milk and salt and cook till the mixture thickens slightly. Add the well-beaten egg-yolks and cook till the eggs are incorporated. Remove from heat and add the grated cheese. Meanwhile beat the egg-whites till they form peaks and fold into the butter mixture. Pour the whole mixture into a well-buttered casserole and place in a pan of hot water. Bake and serve immediately.

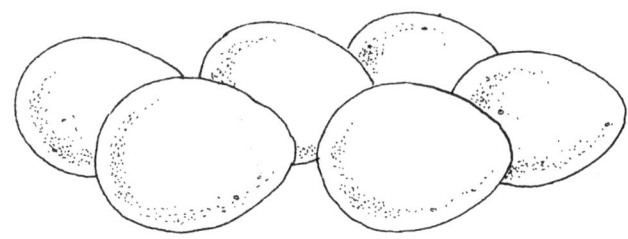

Corn Fritters

Other than sweet corn soup, what can you do with a can of sweet corn? Well, you can make corn fritters with the recipe given below.

Ingredients *(Serves 6)*

- 1 cup self-raising flour
- 2 eggs, lightly beaten
- 310 g can of creamed corn
- 1/2 cup milk

Preparation

Sift flour into a large bowl. Make a well in the centre and blend in the eggs, corn and milk. Keep the mixture aside for about 10 minutes. Heat a shallow pan and brush with melted butter or oil. Drop two teaspoons of the mixture into the pan. When bubbles appear on the surface, turn and cook the other side. Serve on a plate with the herbed cream the recipe of which is given below.

To make herbed cream: Beat 125 g cream cheese. Add 1 tablespoon yoghurt, 1 tablespoon mayonnaise and 2 teaspoons chopped coriander leaves. Mix till creamy and serve with the corn fritters.

Easy Damper

This damper tastes better when spread with extra butter. Forget the extra calories for a day when eating this.

Ingredients *(Serves 8)*
- 4 cups self-raising flour, sifted
- 2 tbsp butter
- 1/2 cup cheese, grated
- 2 tbsp chopped coriander leaves
- 1 cup water
- 1 cup milk

Preparation
Place flour in a large bowl. Rub in the butter till the mixture resembles breadcrumbs. Mix in the cheese, water and milk quickly to form a soft dough. Turn mixture to a lightly floured board and knead lightly. Place in a greased loaf pan. Bake for about 45 minutes or until the loaf sounds hollow when tapped. Serve sliced with extra butter.

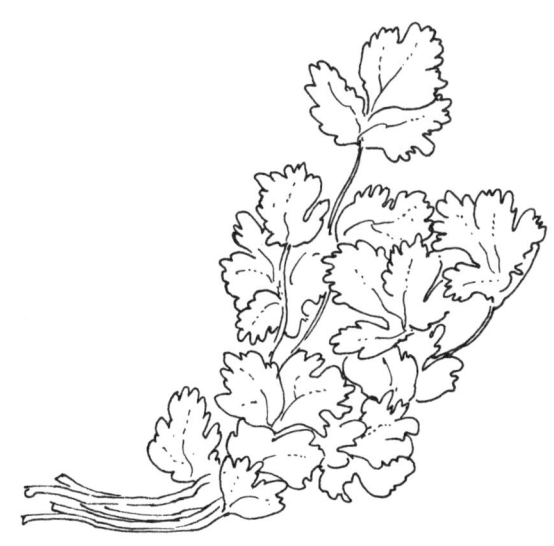

Grilled Tomatoes

This is definitely for the health freak who prefers to be on the safe side.

Ingredients *(Serves 6)*

- 6 large ripe tomatoes
- 2 tbsp olive oil
- 3 cloves garlic, crushed
- 3 slices white bread, crusts removed
- 2 tbsp coriander leaves, chopped
- 1 tbsp spring onions, chopped
- Salt and pepper to taste

Preparation

Cut the tomatoes in half and scoop out most of the pulp and juice. Sprinkle with salt. Leave upside down in a colander to drain for about 1-2 hours and rinse. Mix the olive oil and garlic together and brush both sides of the bread with the mixture to allow it to soften. Chop the bread and leaves together until well-mixed. Press the mixture into the cut tomatoes and drizzle extra olive oil on top. Grill in a pre-heated oven till the top is browned and serve hot.

Macaroni Cheese

Always keep a packet of macaroni in your kitchen. You'll never know when you will need it.

Ingredients *(Serves 4)*

- 1 small packet macaroni, boiled in salted water
- Cheese sauce (as in the cauliflower cheese recipe)
- 3 tbsp breadcrumbs
- 1/4 cup butter or margarine
- Extra grated cheese

Preparation

In a baking dish, arrange the cooked macaroni. Pour the cheese sauce over the macaroni. Cover with extra grated cheese and breadcrumbs. Dot with butter. Bake in a moderately hot oven till the top is slightly brown. Serve.

Onion Rings

This next recipe is not only easy to make but economical as well. Not only is it an all-time snack but an accompaniment to main dishes as well.

Ingredients *(Serves 4)*

- 4 onions, peeled
- 1 cup plain flour, sifted
- 1 cup milk
- 1 egg
- Salt to taste
- Oil for deep-frying

Preparation

Slice the onion thinly and separate into rings. Soak it in the bowl of milk for about an hour to remove any sharpness from the onions. Drain and keep the milk aside for the batter. Beat the egg well, add in the milk, flour and salt. Dip each onion ring into the batter and deep-fry a few at a time. Fry until the rings turn golden brown . Drain well and sprinkle with salt. Serve immediately.

Spicy Potato Rounds

Here is yet another way to make ordinary potatoes turn into an easy-to-make snack. You can avoid the oil too because this is baked.

Ingredients *(Serves 4)*

- 2 cups of mashed potato
- $1\frac{1}{2}$ cups of plain flour
- 1/4 tsp turmeric
- 1/4 tsp garam masala powder
- 1/4 tsp cumin seeds, ground
- 2 cloves garlic, crushed
- 1/4 cup milk
- 60 g melted butter
- 2 tsp coriander leaves, chopped
- Salt to taste

Preparation

Preheat oven to 180° C. Lightly grease and flour the oven trays. Put the mashed potato in a large bowl. Add in the sifted flour and the rest of the ingredients. Stir to form a soft dough. Knead gently for 2 minutes till the dough is smooth. Roll dough between two sheets of plastic wrap or greaseproof paper to 1 cm thickness. Cut into rounds using a plain 10 cm biscuit cutter. Arrange potato rounds on the prepared trays about 3 cms apart. Bake for about 1/2 an hour turning rounds halfway through cooking time.

Spicy Vegetable Fritters

This is the best way to make your children eat vegetables. Use any vegetable that is in season and watch it disappear as soon as it is cooked.

Ingredients *(Serves 6)*

- 250 g plain flour
- 1 tsp ground cumin
- 1 tsp chilli powder
- Salt to taste
- 280 ml water
- 1 tbsp lemon juice
- 1 small cauliflower, broken into small florets
- 250 g mushrooms
- 1 green pepper, cut into 1-inch squares
- 1 potato, cut into 1-inch fingers

Preparation

Put the flour, chilli powder, salt and cumin in a large bowl and gradually add the water and lemon juice, beating well until a smooth batter is formed. Wash the fresh vegetables and dry properly with a clean cloth. Heat oil in a pan. Using a slotted spoon, drop the vegetables a few at a time into the batter, coat completely. Fry the vegetables a few at a time in the hot oil and drain well on paper towels. Serve immediately with tomato or chilli sauce.

Quick Chilli Toast

This recipe is not only unbelievably easy but can be made way ahead of time.

Ingredients *(Serves 6)*

- 12 slices of bread, with crusts removed
- 100 g butter
- 2 cloves garlic
- 1 green chilli, ground
- 1 teaspoon coriander leaves, chopped
- 1/2 tsp pepper

Preparation

Beat the butter, garlic, leaves and pepper with an electric mixer till combined. Spread on the bread slices. Cut the bread diagonally into quarters and place on ungreased oven trays. Bake for about 25 minutes till lightly toasted. These toasts are good for storing in an airtight container.

Rice Cakes

With a little Basmati rice and your imagination, you get not biryani but rice cakes!

Ingredients *(Serves 4)*

- 3 oz biryani rice, cooked
- 1 egg, beaten
- 3 oz grated cheese
- 1 tbsp chopped coriander leaves
- 3 tbsp of flour
- Salt and pepper to taste
- Dry breadcrumbs

Preparation

Mix rice, half the egg, cheese, leaves, salt and pepper together. Add flour to make the mixture stiff. Divide the mixture into balls. Flatten each ball with the palm of your hand to form a flat cake. Dust each cake with flour. Coat with the remaining egg and breadcrumbs. Heat oil in frying pan and shallow fry both sides of each rice cake. Serve hot.

Summer Tomatoes

This is a summer cooler which will keep you not only cool but deliciously healthy as well.

Ingredients *(Serves 3)*

- 6 tomatoes
- 1 tbsp spring onions, chopped
- 4 oz of cheese, grated
- 1 onion, chopped
- Salt and pepper to taste
- 1 cup cooked Basmati rice

Preparation

Remove the core from the bottom of each tomato. Cut a slice from the rounded end of each tomato and scoop out the pulp and seeds with a small teaspoon. Strain out the seeds and use the pulp and juice for the filling. To this, add the rest of the ingredients and mix together thoroughly. Spoon the filling into each of the tomatoes and place them on the serving plates. Top with the reserved tomato slices and serve chilled. You can mix and match the filling ingredients.

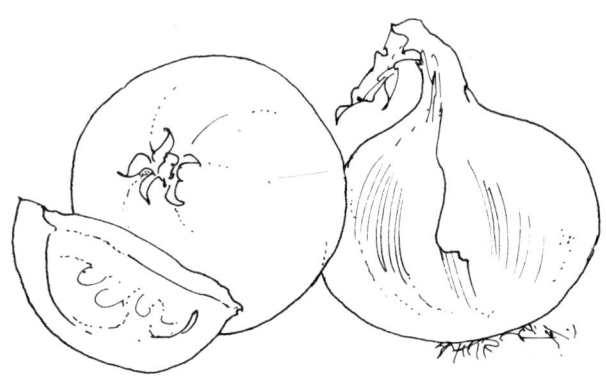

Yummy Potato Rounds

This dish requires no planning ahead. Just take ordinary ingredients from your larder and turn into finger-licking goodies. Just be sure to have lots of tomato sauce around.

Ingredients *(Serves 6)*

- 3/4 kg large old potatoes, peeled and washed
- 2 cups plain flour
- 2 tsp baking powder
- Salt and pepper to taste
- 1 3/4 cups water
- Oil for deep frying

Preparation

Cut the potatoes into thin slices. Dry well. Sift the flour and baking powder together into a bowl. Add the salt and pepper. Gradually add the water till the batter becomes fairly thick. Beat till the batter is smooth with no lumps. Gently coat the potato slices with a little flour first. Then dip each slice into the batter till it is well-coated. Heat the oil and deep-fry a few at a time till it becomes a light golden in colour. Drain. Increase the heat and refry the potato scallops till it becomes golden. Drain again and sprinkle with salt. Serve hot with tomato sauce.

Egg Snacks

Stuffed Eggs

Try these stuffed eggs which reveal a surprise when cut open by your hungry guests.

Ingredients (Serves 2)

- 4 hard-boiled eggs
- 1/2 cup mushrooms, chopped finely
- 1 oz spring onions, chopped
- 1 cup white sauce
- 1 tbsp tomato sauce
- 1/2 cup cheese, grated

Preparation

Cut eggs in half, lengthwise. Remove the yolks, mash and mix with the mushrooms, spring onions, salt and pepper. Stuff back into the egg-white halves. Mix the white sauce and tomato sauce together. Arrange the eggs in a shallow baking dish. Cover with the white sauce mixture. Sprinkle cheese on top and bake in a moderate oven till the cheese melts.

Egg-White Cheese Balls

This is enough to serve six people. Double the quantity and you will have enough to serve a party.

Ingredients (Serves 6)

- 2 oz cheese, grated
- 1 oz flour
- 1 egg, separated
- Salt and pepper to taste
- Oil for deep-frying

Preparation

Mix the cheese, flour, salt and pepper with the yolk of the egg. Whip the egg-white stiffly. Stir lightly into the cheese mixture. Drop teaspoonfuls into hot oil. Cook till golden brown. Serve hot with tomato sauce.

Quick Sandwich

What do you do when guests pop in unexpectedly? Try this quick snack with a hot cup of tea, and your guests will be more than satisfied.

Ingredients *(Serves 3)*

- 6 slices of white bread
- 50 g butter
- Parsley for garnish

For the filling

- 2 eggs, boiled
- 25 g butter
- 2 tomatoes, sliced thinly

Preparation

Mash the eggs with the butter and season well with salt and pepper. Butter the bread on one side and spread the filling on it. Top with the sliced tomato and cover with a second buttered slice of bread. Trim the crust and cut into any shape desired. Repeat with the rest of the slices of bread. Serve garnished with parsley or mint leaves.

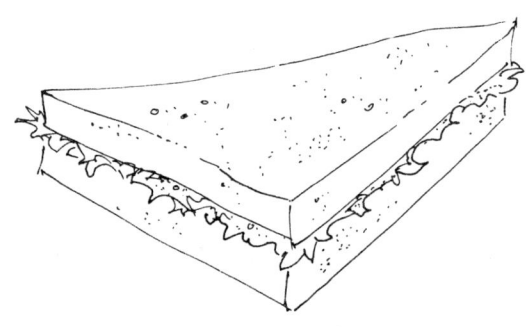

Egg in Potato Nest

As the name suggests, the next recipe will definitely keep people guessing!!

Ingredients *(Serves 2)*

- 2 eggs
- 3 potatoes, boiled and mashed
- 25 g butter
- 2 tbsp milk
- Salt and pepper to taste

Preparation

In a bowl, add the salt, pepper and butter to the mashed potatoes. Mix well. Add the milk gradually and mix till creamy. Divide the mixture equally into 2 heatproof bowls and shape so that there is a hollow in the centre, like a nest. Break an egg into each of the bowls and place the bowls in a baking tray half filled with water. Bake till the eggs set. Serve garnished with a little pepper and grated cheese.

Aberdeen Eggs

Surprise your guests with this snack. Covered with breadcrumbs, no one will suspect what is inside!

Ingredients *(Serves 4)*

- 4 hard-boiled eggs, shelled
- 1/2 cup breadcrumbs, seasoned with salt and pepper
- Flour, to coat
- 1 egg, beaten
- 12 oz chicken, minced
- Oil for deep-frying

Preparation

Cover each egg firmly with the chicken meat. Roll in the flour and then the egg. Roll in breadcrumbs and chill till ready to fry. Deep-fry till golden brown and serve with salad.

Variation: You can substitute the chicken meat with sausage meat.

Steamed Egg Snack

A snack with a difference, this snack is not only easy but nutritious as well. The prawns make it delicious.

Ingredients (Serves 4)

- 3 eggs, beaten
- 1/4 cup shallots, sliced
- 2 tbsp oil
- $1\frac{1}{2}$ cups water
- 20 g prawns, shelled and chopped
- 1/4 tsp sugar
- Salt and pepper to taste

For the garnish
- 1 stalk spring onion, chopped
- 1 tbsp reserved oil from frying shallots

Preparation

Heat oil in a pan and lightly brown shallots. Drain and keep aside. Reserve the shallot oil for garnish. In the beaten eggs, add the salt, pepper, sugar, water and prawns. Mix and pour into a heatproof dish. Steam over boiling water for about 10-15 minutes till the custard has just set. Sprinkle the garnish ingredients on top and serve hot.

Eggs Florentine

Easy to make in a hurry and very nutritious too.

Ingredients *(Serves 2)*

- 1 cup spinach
- 2 tsp butter
- Salt and pepper to taste
- 4-6 hard boiled eggs (cut into quarters)
- Cheese sauce (recipe given below)

Preparation

Cook the spinach and drain. Make sure it is free from water. Chop it finely and add the butter and seasoning. Arrange the spinach in a pretty dish. Place the eggs on top. Cover with the cheese sauce and serve.

Cheese Sauce: In a saucepan, put 2 cups of milk, 1 cup of grated cheese, salt and pepper, 1 tsp mustard and tbsp flour. Heat gently stirring till the cheese dissolves. Cook till thick and serve as directed.

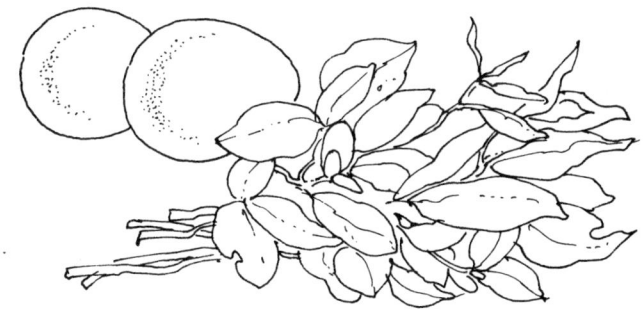

Light Spanish Frittata

This snack is easy and a real treat too!

Ingredients (Serves 6)

- 6 eggs
- 2 tbsp butter
- 1 potato, peeled and sliced thinly
- 1 onion, thinly sliced
- 1 tomato, peeled and chopped
- 1 strip of bacon, trimmed of fat and chopped
- Salt and pepper to taste

Preparation

Heat butter in a pan and sauté the onion and potato till tender. Add the tomato and bacon. When cooked, remove from pan. In a bowl, whisk the eggs with salt and pepper. Pour over the potato mixture and shake the pan gently so that it does not stick. When the edges begin to set, place a large plate over the pan and flip the pan over so that the frittata is turned over. Slide back into the heated pan and cook the other side for about 2 minutes. Divide into six and serve with toasted bread spread with butter.

Omelette Pizza

So you thought pizza could only be made with flour. Well try this and see how wrong you were.

Ingredients *(Serves 2)*

- 6 eggs, beaten
- 100 g cheese
- 4 mushrooms, sliced
- 1 capsicum, chopped
- 4 tomatoes, peeled and chopped
- 2 tbsp tomato paste
- Parsley, chopped (optional)
- 2 tsps butter or margarine
- Salt and pepper to taste

Preparation

Add the tomatoes, parsley, tomato paste, salt and pepper to the eggs and mix well. Heat 2 teaspoons of butter or margarine in a frying pan. Pour the omelette mixture and spread the mushroom, capsicum and cheese over the omelette. Cover the pan and let the omelette cook for about 5-10 minutes. Serve hot.

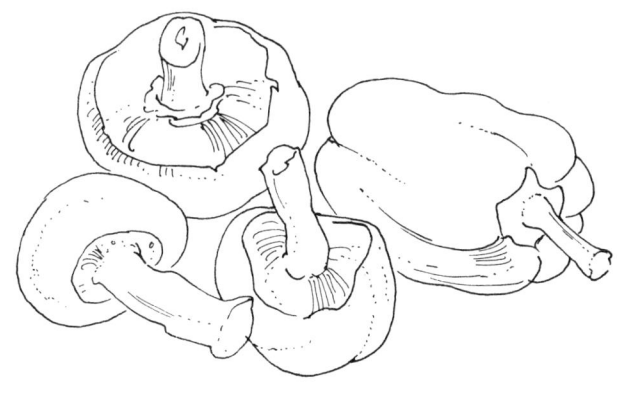

Yummy Fluffy Omelettes

Any time is good time for omelettes. These yummy fluffy omelettes will definitely stay on top of your omelette list.

Ingredients *(Serves 3)*

- 8 eggs, separated
- 1/2 cup flour
- 1/4 cup water
- Salt and pepper to taste,
- 1/2 tsp cream of tartar
- 4 tbsp butter
- $1\frac{1}{2}$ cups milk
- 1/2 cup grated cheese
- Butter for frying

Preparation

Beat egg-yolks with 1/4 cup of flour and 1/4 cup water. Add salt and pepper. Beat till thick and creamy. Beat the egg-whites with cream of tartar till stiff but not dry. Fold egg-yolk mixture gently into the beaten egg-whites. Pile the mixture into 2 well- buttered cake pans. Bake at 350 for 15 minutes. During this time, prepare the cheese sauce. Melt butter in a pan. Add the remaining 1/4 cup of flour, salt and milk. Cook until slightly thickened. Add cheese and stir. Place 1 baked layer on a serving plate and top with half of the cheese sauce. Place the second layer on top and cover with the remaining sauce. Use 2 forks to cut the omelette since it is light. Serve immediately.

Seafood Snacks

Cold Prawn Balls

This is not only easy to make but can be kept away in the fridge for almost a day in advance and served cold.

Ingredients *(Serves 3)*

- 1 cup cooked prawns, chopped
- 2 hard-boiled eggs, chopped
- 2 tbsp cheese, grated
- 2 tbsp mayonnaise
- 1 tbsp lemon juice
- 1 tbsp chopped parsley or coriander leaves
- Salt and pepper to taste

Preparation

In a bowl, mix the prawns, eggs, cheese, mayonnaise, lemon juice, salt and pepper well. Form teaspoonfuls of the mixture into little balls. Roll in the chopped leaves. Chill for a minimum of 2 hours and serve.

Sardine Sandwich

Always keep a tin of sardines in your larder for a quick tasty snack which will go a long way.

Ingredients *(Serves 3)*

- 6 slices of bread
- 25 g butter

For the filling

- 2 sardines, drained and mashed
- 1 small onion, chopped finely
- Juice of 1 lime
- 1/2 cucumber, cut into thin slices
- 2 tomatoes, sliced thinly

Preparation

Butter the bread. To the mashed sardines, add the onion and lime juice. Spread the filling on each buttered bread slice. Top with cucumber and tomato and a second slice of bread. Trim the crust and cut into triangles. Serve garnished with extra cucumber and tomato slices.

Bread Squares

Try these bread squares for a change. And forget the calories for a day.

Ingredients (Serves 4)

- 4 slices of bread
- 125 g prawns, cleaned and chopped finely
- 2 small onions, chopped finely
- Salt and pepper to taste
- 1 egg, beaten
- Oil for deep-frying

Preparation

Cut each slice of bread into 4 squares. In a small bowl, mix the prawns, onion, salt and pepper. Divide this mixture equally and spread on each of the 16 squares of bread. Heat the oil. Dip each bread square into the beaten egg and fry till golden brown. Drain on kitchen paper. Serve hot garnished with cucumber slices and chopped red chilli.

Fish Loaf

Serve this loaf with a salad and some lemon wedges and it is sure to be a filling snack.

Ingredients (Serves 5)

- 1/2 kg of fish, minced
- 1 packet of mushroom soup About 2 cups of breadcrumbs
- 1 onion, chopped finely
- 2 eggs, separated
- 1 tbsp coriander leaves, chopped
- 1 tbsp lemon juice
- Salt and pepper

Preparation

Preheat the oven. In a mixing bowl, stir in the soup powder, fish, onion, egg-yolks, crumbs, lemon juice, coriander leaves, salt and pepper. Mix well. Meanwhile beat the egg-whites till stiff and fold into the fish mixture. Spread into the tin and bake for almost an hour. Serve sliced.

Fish Sausage

Try these fish sausages for a change. Your family will love the taste and ask for more.

Ingredients *(Serves 4)*

- 1/2 kg of boneless fish, minced
- 2 tbsp green shallots, chopped
- 1 carrot, grated
- 1 tbsp lemon juice
- 1/2 cup breadcrumbs
- 2 tbsp chopped parsley, optional
- 2 eggs, lightly beaten
- Plain flour
- 3 tbsp oil
- 20 g butter

Preparation

Combine the shallots, carrot, parsley, lemon juice, breadcrumbs, eggs and fish in a bowl. Shape a little of the mixture into sausages and toss in flour. Heat the oil and the butter in a frying pan. Add the sausages and cook over medium heat for about 10 minutes till cooked and well-browned. Serve hot with sauce.

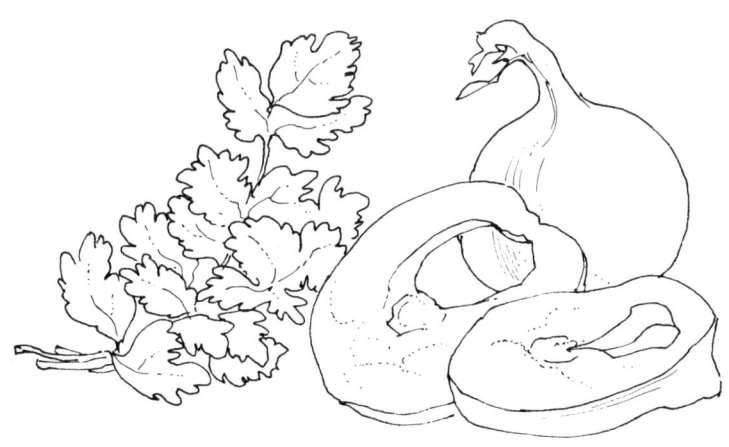

Fish and Tomato Loaf

This loaf will be a surprise because your guests will never guess the surprise filling inside!!

Ingredients *(Serves 4)*

- 1 small loaf of bread
- 1 cooked potato, cut into cubes
- 1/2 kg of fish, cooked and minced
- 2 tbsp shallots, chopped
- 1/4 cup cream
- 1 egg

Preparation

Cut 1/3rd from the top of bread and remove the crumbs from inside the loaf, leaving the crust 1 cm thick. Keep the crumbs for later use.
Combine the fish, potato, shallots, cream and egg and fill the crust. Replace the top of the loaf and wrap tightly in foil. Bake for about 1/2 an hour to 45 minutes. Serve with tomato sauce.

Crumbed Cheese Fish

Made with common ingredients, this dish is best made just before serving.

Ingredients *(Serves 4)*

- 1/2 kg fish, cut into strips
- 1 egg, beaten
- 2 tbsp milk
- 1 cup breadcrumbs
- 1/4 cup cheese, grated plain flour
- Oil for deep-frying

Preparation

Season the fish strips with salt and pepper. Toss the fish strips in flour. Dip into the combined egg and milk, then combined cheese and breadcrumbs. Deep-fry in hot oil till golden brown. Serve hot with sauce.

Toasted Seafood Sandwich

Get your sandwich maker ready for this next delight!!

Ingredients *(Serves 4)*

- 10 slices of bread, spread evenly with butter
- 1/4 kg prawns, shelled and cooked
- 1 cup cheese, grated
- 1 tbsp tomato paste
- 1 tbsp green shallots, chopped

Preparation

Combine remaining ingredients and spread 5 slices of bread with this mixture. Top with the remaining slices and cook in a sandwich maker till golden brown. Serve hot.

Deep-Fried King Prawn

Don't know what to do with that extra kilo of king prawns? Try this and feast with delight.

Ingredients *(Serves 8)*

- I kg king prawns, shelled and deveined, with the tails intact
- Plain flour
- 1/2 cup oats
- 1/2 cup almonds, chopped
- 1 egg
- 1 tbsp milk
- Oil for deep frying

Preparation

Dust prawns with the flour and dip in the combined egg and milk. Mix the oats and almonds together. Press prawns into this mixture and refrigerate for 1/2 an hour. Deep-fry in hot oil till golden brown. Sprinkle salt and serve with mayonnaise.

Chilli Prawn Croquettes

Freeze these after the rolling in the breadcrumbs and you always have a snack in hand.

Ingredients *(Serves 2)*

- 1 cup prawns, peeled, deveined and minced
- 1/2 cup celery, chopped
- 1 egg, beaten
- 3 tbsp butter
- 3 tbsp flour
- 3/4 cup milk
- 1 tsp chilli powder
- 3/4 cup breadcrumbs
- Flour
- Salt and pepper to taste
- Oil for deep-frying

Preparation

Melt butter. Add the flour and stir till smooth. Add milk and bring to the boil gradually. Stir to make sure no lumps form. Cook for about 3 minutes. Add the prawns, celery and seasoning. Chill in the refrigerator till firm. Divide the mixture into 12 pieces according to preference and shape into croquettes. Coat each piece with flour. Then dip in the egg followed by the breadcrumbs. Fry croquettes in hot oil till golden brown. Serve hot.

Butterfly Prawns

What do butterfly prawns look like? Try this and see.

Ingredients

- 1/2 kg big prawns, peeled and deveined
- 1 egg, beaten
- 1 tbsp milk
- Seasoned flour
- Breadcrumbs
- Oil for deep-frying

Preparation

Cut each prawn right through to resemble a butterfly. Dip in the flour, then in egg mixed with milk. Dip each prawn firmly in the breadcrumbs. Till serving time these can be left in the refrigerator. When needed, fry the prawns in hot oil and serve hot with lots of tomato sauce. An easy snack but really tasty.

Pinwheel Sandwiches

Instead of the usual sandwiches, try these pinwheels for a change.

Ingredients (Serves 4)

- 4 slices fresh bread
- 1 oz butter
- 1/2 cup boneless fish, boiled and minced
- 1 tsp lemon juice
- Salt and pepper to taste
- 1/2 cup paneer, crumbled

Preparation

Cut off the crusts of the bread. Mix all the ingredients and spread on the buttered slices.
Roll up each slice of bread and wrap tightly in greaseproof paper or foil. Chill. Remove paper and cut into 1/2 inch slices. Serve garnished with parsley or coriander leaves.

Kofta Fish Balls

These little balls can be served hot with cocktail sticks and a variety of dips.

Ingredients *(Serves 4)*

- 400 g cooked white fish
- 1 onion, minced
- 1 tsp coriander powder
- 1 tsp turmeric powder
- 1/2 tsp cumin, ground
- 1 tsp ginger, ground
- 1 tbsp lime juice
- 2 eggs, beaten
- Salt to taste
- Oil for frying
- Breadcrumbs

Preparation

Process all the ingredients together except eggs, breadcrumbs and oil. Form into small balls and roll in the beaten eggs and then in the breadcrumbs. Deep-fry till golden brown. Drain on kitchen towels.

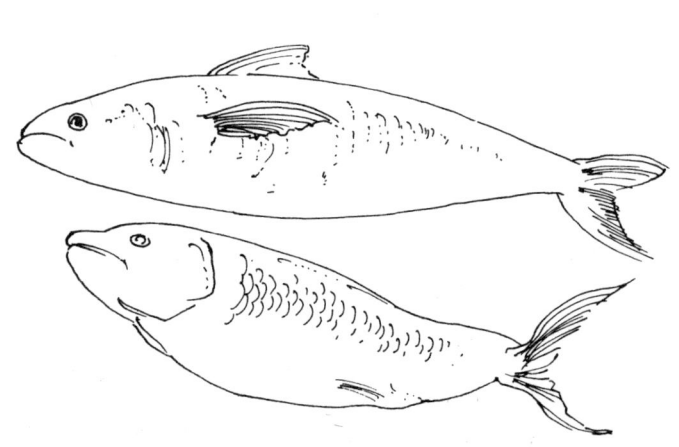

Crabmeat Balls

Now you know what to do when crabs are in season.

Ingredients *(Serves 4)*

- 1/2 kg crabmeat, chopped finely
- 4 slices of bread, crusts removed
- 15 g butter
- 1 tbsp flour
- 1/2 green pepper, minced
- 1 tsp green chilli, chopped
- 1 spring onion, finely chopped
- 1 tbsp coriander leaves
- Salt to taste
- 2 eggs, beaten
- Dry breadcrumbs
- Oil to deep-fry

Preparation

Combine the crabmeat with the fresh breadcrumbs and keep aside. Melt the butter in a pan and add the flour. Take off the heat. Stir in the milk and return to a moderate heat. Bring to the boil, stirring constantly. Stir this sauce into the crabmeat and breadcrumb mixture. Add the spring onion, chillies and the coriander leaves. Season with salt and let it cool completely. Shape the crabmeat into 1-inch balls with floured hands. Coat with the beaten egg and then coat with the dry breadcrumbs. Fry the balls in hot oil, 6 at a time till they turn golden brown. Turn balls occasionally. Drain on paper towels and sprinkle lightly with salt. Serve hot.

Fish Croquettes

Try this out for your kids and they will be constantly asking for more. You might need to make more than the quantity specified.

Ingredients *(Serves 4)*

- 1/4 kg boneless fish, like tuna or salmon
- 1 tsp curry powder
- 1 onion, chopped
- 1 tbsp lemon juice
- 1 tbsp chopped coriander leaves
- 2 eggs
- Breadcrumbs
- Oil for deep frying

To Make White Sauce
- 90 g butter
- 3/4 cup plain flour
- 3 cups milk
- Salt and pepper to taste

Preparation

To make the white sauce: Melt the butter over low heat. Remove from heat and stir in the flour till smooth. Return to the heat and cook a few more minutes. Remove from heat and gradually stir in the milk. Return to heat and stir till the milk boils. Reduce heat and simmer for another 3 minutes. Season with salt and pepper.

To make the croquettes: To chopped fish add the curry powder, lemon juice, onion, coriander leaves. Mix this mixture into the white sauce. Mix well. Spread this on to a shallow tray and refrigerate till firm. Then mould the mixture to croquette shapes of 1 inch by 2 inches. Dip first in the beaten eggs then press firmly into the breadcrumb mixture. Refrigerate for another 1 hour. Deep fry till golden brown for a few minutes. Drain and serve hot.

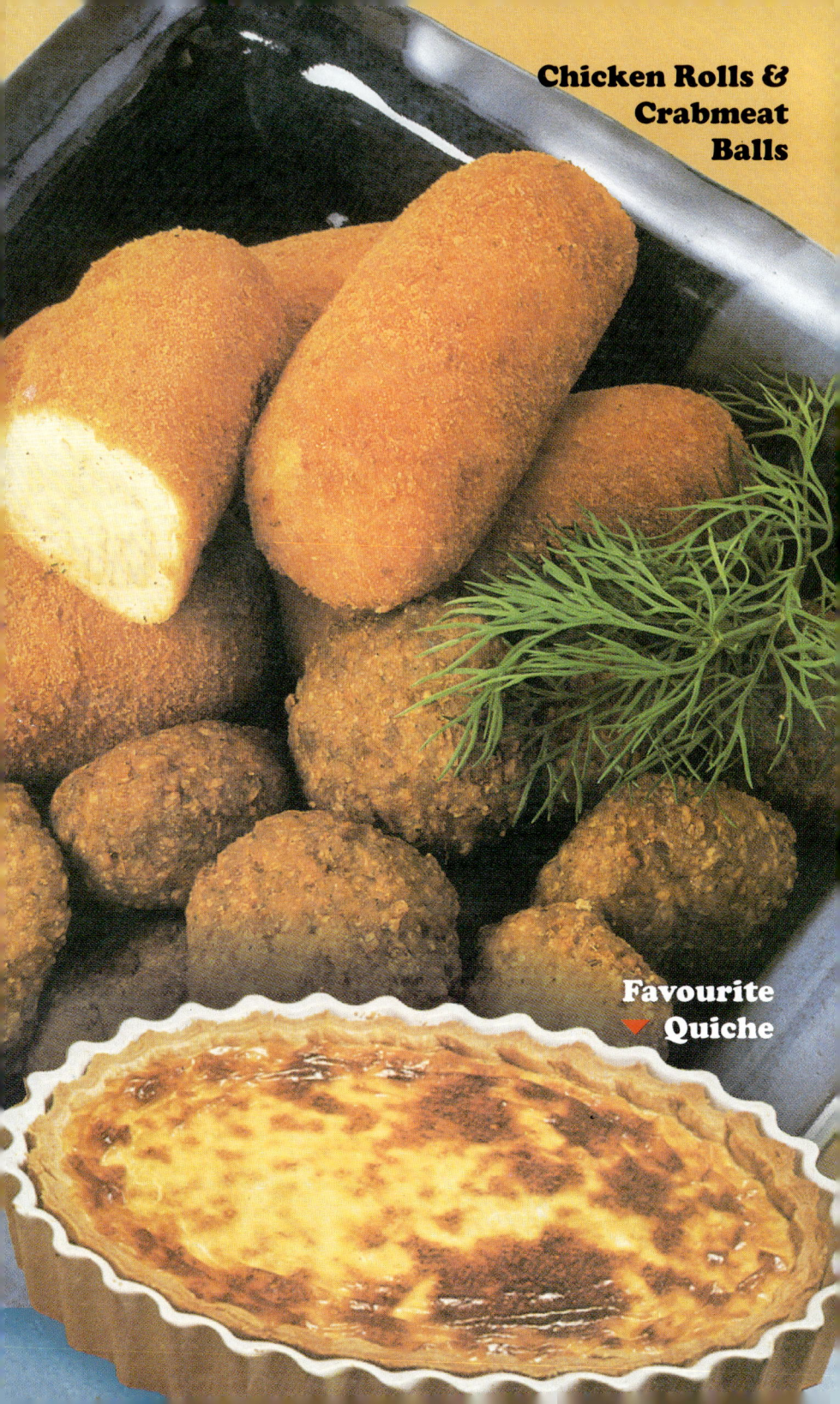

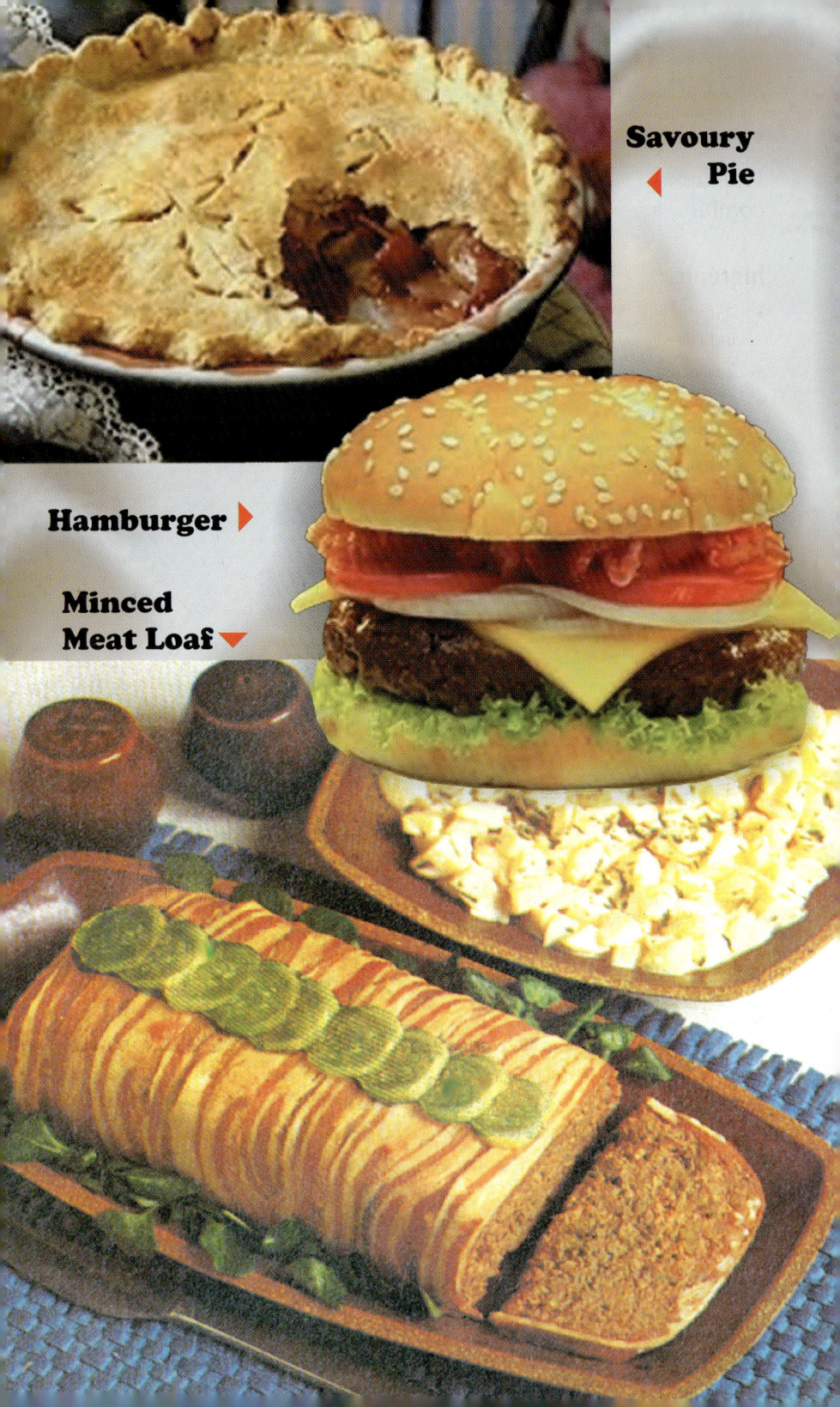

Fish Pie

Watch how simple ingredients like fish and potatoes can combine together to become an exotic pie.

Ingredients *(Serves 6)*

- 750 g white fish pieces, cooked in boiling water
- 2 carrots, sliced
- 60 g (2 oz) butter
- 1 onion, chopped
- 2 tbsp curry powder
- 3 tbsp flour
- 2 oz (60g) green peas, cooked
- 750 g potatoes, peeled and cooked in salted water
- 1 tbsp coriander leaves or parsley chopped
- 5 tbsp milk
- 2 oz cheese, grated
- 1 egg-yolk

Preparation

Reserve the water in which the fish was cooked. Melt butter in a saucepan. Stir in the onion and curry powder. Fry till the onion becomes soft. Stir in the flour over a low heat. Remove pan from heat and add the fish stock (about $1^1/_2$ cups) gently till well-blended. Add the carrots, peas, salt and pepper. Simmer for 2 minutes. Add the fish pieces with the leaves. Pour into an 8-inch pie-dish. Mash the potatoes well and season with salt and pepper. Add in the milk and cheese. Mix well. Spread this mashed potato mixture over the fish filling and make a design on top with a fork. Beat egg-yolk with a little water and brush over the potatoes. Bake in a moderate oven till the top turns golden brown.

Fish Tempura

If you want to go Japanese, this is the best way to do it. Tempura is definitely on their favourites list.

Ingredients *(Serves 6)*

- 300 g of firm, white fish, cut into 2 x 1 inch strips
- 6 large prawns
- 30 g plain flour for dusting
- 120 ml (4 fl oz) of iced water
- 4 oz plain flour
- Oil

Preparation

Shell the prawns leaving the tails intact. Dry the fish and dust both the prawns and fish with flour. Beat the water and egg-yolk together. Add the 4 ozs of flour and mix well. Dip each piece of fish in the batter and deep-fry in hot oil, a few pieces at a time. Drain and put on paper towels. Repeat the same procedure with the prawns. Serve hot with the sauce below.

Sauce: Mix together 2 tbsp soy sauce, juice of 2 lemons and 2 tsps of vinegar and 2 chopped green chillies.

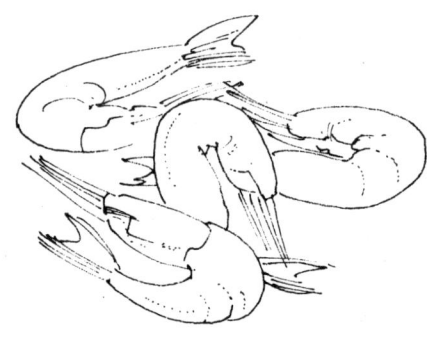

PRAWN COCKTAIL

This is very easy to make and a favourite. Use as much prawns as you like. Don't forget to make extra dressing.

Ingredients (Serves 2)

- 1 cup cooked prawns or shrimps
- Lettuce leaves
- Dressing (recipe given below)
- Lemon slices for garnish

Dressing

- 1 egg-yolk
- Salt and pepper to taste
- 1 tsp sugar
- 1 tbsp vinegar
- 1 tbsp warm water
- 2 tbsp tomato ketchup
- 1 tsp Worcestershire sauce
- 2 tbsp olive oil

Preparation

Shred the lettuce. In a salad bowl, or individual glasses, put in some lettuce. Top with the prawns mixed with the dressing. Garnish with lemon slices.

Dressing: Put egg-yolk and seasonings in bowl and mix. Beat in the vinegar gradually, then add the warm water. Beat in the oil, a drop at a time till the mixture thickens. Stir in the tomato ketchup and the Worcestershire sauce. If you are using an electric blender, blend the egg-yolk, vinegar, water and seasonings in the blender. Then add the oil.

Prawn Pastry Puffs

Ingredients *(Serves 6)*

- 90 g butter
- 90 ml water
- 90 g flour, sieved
- 4 eggs, beaten
- 45 g butter
- 45 g flour
- 280 ml milk
- 180 g or 6 oz peeled prawns, chopped
- 7 hard-boiled eggs, chopped
- 1 tsp chopped herbs
- Pinch of nutmeg
- Salt and pepper to taste

Preparation

Put the butter and water in a pan. Bring to the boil over a medium heat. Tip in the flour all at once and beat until the mixture is smooth and leaves the sides of the pan clean. Remove from the heat and leave to cool slightly. Add the eggs gradually to the flour mixture beating vigorously till the mixture forms a shiny, smooth paste. Grease a baking sheet and drop teaspoonfuls of the mixture onto it spaced well-apart. Bake for about 25 minutes in a moderate oven till the puffs are firm to the touch and golden brown. Melt the remaining butter in a pan and stir in the remaining flour. Blend in the milk gradually, beating well. Bring milk to the boil. While stirring add the remaining ingredients. Cut the pastry puffs almost in half through the middle and fill with the prawn and egg mixture.

Chicken Snacks

Cheese Canapes

Bread is indispensable around the house. This is one of the reasons why.

Ingredients *(Serves 4)*

- 8 slices white bread
- 2 tbsp butter, melted
- 2 egg-whites, beaten stiffly
- 1/2 cup cheese, grated
- 1 tbsp spring onion, chopped
- 3 rashers bacon, chopped (optional)
- Salt and pepper to taste

Preparation

Cut the bread diagonally into 16 pieces. Toast on one side and brush the other side with butter. Mix the rest of the ingredients except the bacon together. Spoon mixture on the buttered side of the bread and sprinkle the bacon on top. Grill till the bacon turns brown and the cheese melts. Serve hot. For vegetarians, substitute the bacon with green pepper cut into strips.

Vegetable and Rice Custard

You've heard of caramel custard but have you heard of the next dish?

Ingredients

- 1/2 cup cooked chicken, chopped
- 1 tbsp oil
- 2 carrots, chopped
- 1/2 cup celery, chopped
- 1/2 cup cucumber, chopped
- 2/3 cup raw rice, cooked to get about 2 cups of white rice
- 1/2 cup thick cream
- 4 eggs, beaten lightly
- 1/2 cup cheese, grated
- 2 tbsp coriander leaves, chopped
- 1 tbsp parsley, chopped (optional)
- Salt and pepper to taste

Preparation

Grease a square 23 cm pan. Heat the oil and fry carrots, celery, cucumber and the chicken. When the carrots are cooked, combine the rest of the ingredients and mix well. Spread mixture in the prepared pan and bake for about 1/2 an hour or more till the custard sets.

Almond Cream Dip

Always keep crackers or potato chips on hand for a quick snack.

Ingredients *(Serves 2)*

- 1 cup fish or chicken, minced
- 1/2 cup chopped green pepper
- 1/4 cup onion, chopped
- 1 tsp Worcestershire sauce
- 2 tbsp mayonnaise
- 1 tbsp almonds, toasted
- 1/4 cup cream, beaten till thick crackers
- Potato chips or bread cut into circles

Preparation

Mix the first five ingredients together. Add the beaten cream. Garnish with the almonds and serve with crackers, chips or toasted bread cut in fancy shapes.

Chicken and Cucumber Double Decker

How about some light sandwiches to face a hot day?

Ingredients *(Serves 3)*

- 9 slices of bread, buttered
- 12 slices thinly sliced cucumber
- Salt and pepper to taste
- 1 cup cooked chicken, diced

Preparation

Butter each slice of bread well. Place the 4 cucumber slices on 3 bread slices. Layer each separately with a second slice of bread. Spread chicken on this and cover with the third slice of bread. Slice each triple sandwich diagonally to get 6 sandwiches.

Grilled Chicken

Instead of fried chicken, try this grilled chicken for a change.

Ingredients *(Serves 4)*

- 4 chicken breast fillets
- 1 cup orange juice
- 2 tsps orange rind, grated
- 1 tsp chicken stock powder
- 1 tbsp chopped coriander leaves
- 1/2 tsp curry powder
- 1/2 tsp nutmeg, ground
- Salt and pepper to taste

Preparation

Mix all the marinade ingredients together and stir well. Add the chicken and coat well with the marinade. Cover and keep in the fridge for 2-3 hours. Take out the chicken and grill turning frequently. Keep brushing the chicken with the marinade mixture. Serve as high protein healthy snack.

Easy Chicken Wings

Try this out and you will see why it is so easy.

Ingredients *(Serves 5)*
- 10 chicken wings
- 2 tbsp lemon juice
- 1/3 cup soya sauce
- 1 1/2 tsp ginger, ground
- 2 tbsp honey
- 2 tbsp tomato sauce

Preparation

Marinate the chicken in the mixture of lemon juice, soya sauce and ginger for about 3 hours. Drain the wings but save the marinade. In a cup, mix the honey, tomato sauce and the remaining marinade. Grill the wings for about 5-10 minutes after brushing the wings with the honey mixture. Turn over and brush with more of the honey mixture. Grill till cooked and serve hot.

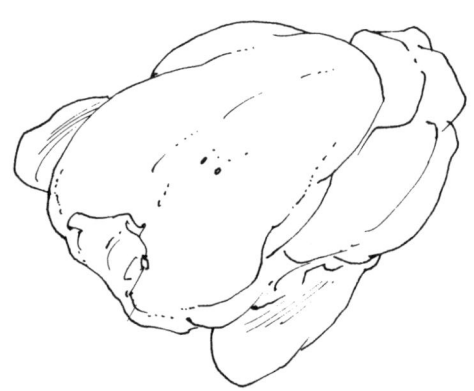

Chicken and Potato Scones

A good mixture of protein and carbohydrate, this snack will give your children all the energy they need.

Ingredients *(Serves 4)*

- 270 g plain flour sifted with 3 tsp baking powder
- 90 g butter
- 90 g chicken, cooked
- 1/4 cup coriander leaves, chopped
- 180 g potatoes, cooked and mashed
- 1/4 cup milk
- Salt and pepper to taste

For the glaze
- Beat together 1 egg-yolk with 1 tsp of milk

Preparation

In a bowl, rub butter into the sifted flour with a pastry knife or cutter till the mixture resembles breadcrumbs. Stir in the rest of the ingredients and mix till it becomes a soft dough. Turn onto a lightly floured board and roll out on a sheet of plastic wrap to about 2 cms thick. Cut into desired shapes with the cookie cutter and place on a greased tray. Bake for about 20 minutes till golden brown. Remove from oven and brush scones immediately with the egg-glaze. Serve hot.

American Fried Chicken Wings

Have paper napkins handy for this next finger licking treat.

Ingredients *(Serves 6)*
- 12 chicken wings
- 2 tbsp oil
- 2 cloves garlic, crushed
- 1 tbsp Worcestershire sauce
- 1 tbsp tomato ketchup
- 1 tsp sugar
- 2 tsp mustard sauce
- 1 tbsp lemon juice
- Seasoned flour
- Oil for frying

Preparation

Mix the oil, the sauces and the ketchup, garlic, sugar, salt and lemon juice. Make cuts on the chicken and mix the marinade into the chicken. Put in a polythene bag and keep for several hours. It can also be refrigerated overnight for the flavours to blend.

Roll the chicken wings in flour and fry till well-browned all over. Serve hot.

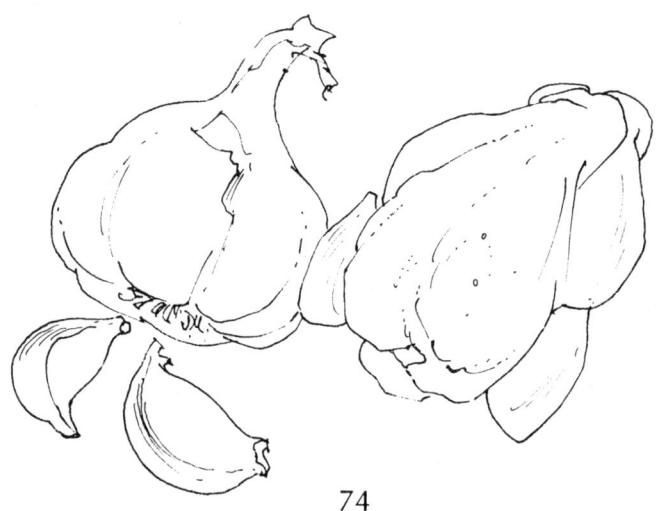

Crusty Rice Pizza

Snacks with left-over rice always come in handy because left-over rice is inevitable in every household. Serve the rice as a pizza... what an idea!!

Ingredients (Serves 3)

- 3 cups rice, cooked
- 1 cup cheese, grated
- 1 tsp garlic, mashed
- 2 eggs, beaten
- 1 cup tomato sauce
- 1/2 cup mushrooms, sliced
- 1/2 cup cooked chicken, minced
- 1/2 cup green pepper (capsicum) thinly sliced

Preparation

In a bowl, mix the rice, eggs and cheese well. Put this mixture into a flat frying pan and spread out the mixture to cover the base of the pan. Cover and cook for at least 15 minutes. When it becomes brown and crusty, spread tomato sauce mixed with salt, pepper and garlic on the top of the crusty base. Top with the chicken, green pepper and mushrooms and sprinkle with cheese. Cover and cook a further 10 minutes. Uncover and cook another 5-10 minutes. Serve garnished with chopped spring onions.

Chicken Cakes

What? Cakes made with chicken? This will certainly be something different but yummy.

Ingredients *(Serves 3)*

- 400 g minced chicken
- 1 onion peeled and chopped
- 1 carrot, peeled and chopped
- 1/2 tsp sugar
- 1 tbsp cornflour
- 2 tsp soya sauce
- Salt and pepper to taste

Preparation

Mix all the ingredients together and leave the meat mixture aside to marinate for at least half an hour. Heat oil in a frying pan. Shape the meat mixture into balls and flatten them a little with your palm. Gently slide the cakes into hot oil and fry until golden brown. Serve hot with chilli sauce.

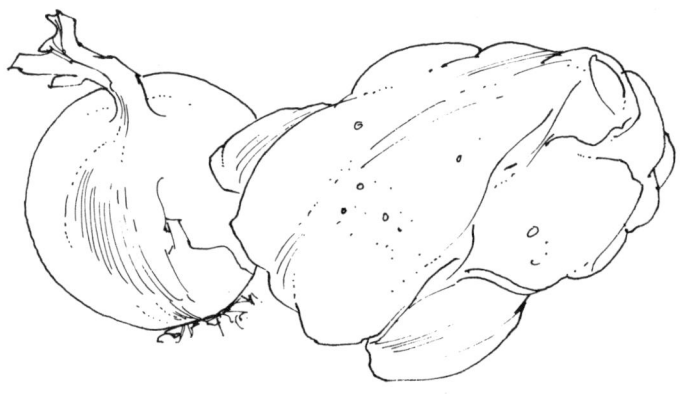

Chicken Pastry

When you have extra time on your hands this pastry is definitely worth the extra effort.

Ingredients *(Serves 4)*

- 2 cups flour
- 1 tsp baking powder
- 120 g (4 oz) pastry margarine
- 45 g butter

For Filling

- 2 cups chicken meat, seasoned with salt and pepper
- 1 cucumber, diced
- 3 tbsp mayonnaise
- Salt and pepper to taste
- 1 tomato to garnish

Preparation

Sift the flour and baking powder into a bowl. Rub in the margarine till the mixture resembles breadcrumbs. Mix in the butter along with cold water as required to make the dough soft. Cover dough with a dry cloth and keep aside for half an hour. Roll out dough on a floured board to about 1 cm in thickness. Divide mentally into 3 equal parts and fold the 1st part over to the centre. Now fold over the centre to the 3 rd part. It is now in 3 layers. Repeat the rolling and folding procedure 2 more times. Divide the pastry into 2 for easier handling. Roll out into circles and put into ungreased patty tins and bake in a hot oven for about 20 minutes. When done, remove from tins and cool on a wire rack. Fill with the chicken stuffing and garnish with thin tomato strips.

Method for the filling: Cut the chicken into small pieces. In a bowl put the chicken, cucumber and mayonnaise and mix well. Add the salt and pepper. Then proceed as above. Chicken can also be substituted with prawns and other vegetables.

Crepe Delight

Try these crepes for a real delight. The best part: You can make these and store in the refrigerator up to a day ahead.

Ingredients *(Serves 4)*

- 1 cup plain flour, sifted
- 3 eggs, lightly beaten
- $1\frac{1}{4}$ cups milk
- 2 tbsp oil

For Filling

- 300 g chicken, cooked and chopped
- 3 eggs, hard-boiled and chopped
- 1/2 cup mayonnaise

Preparation

In a bowl, stir in the milk, eggs and oil into the flour. Beat until the mixture becomes smooth. Pour 2 tbsp of batter into a greased pan and cook until it turns slightly brown. Turn and cook the other side also. Repeat with the remaining batter. Place about 2 teaspoons of filling at one end of each of the crepes and roll up. Fold in the sides to form a parcel. Grease an ovenproof dish and place the parcels in and bake covered in a moderate oven for about 35 minutes. Serve hot with a dish of cool yoghurt.

Method for the filling: Combine all the ingredients into a bowl and mix well.

Chicken Rolls

What do you do with chicken and bread? Make chicken rolls, of course!

Ingredients *(Serves 4)*

- 300 g cooked chicken, minced
- 2 cups breadcrumbs
- 2 tsps lemon juice
- 2 eggs
- 1 onion, chopped
- 1 tsp coriander leaves, chopped
- Dry breadcrumbs
- Salt and pepper to taste
- Oil for deep-frying

Preparation

Mix the chicken, lemon juice, salt, pepper, breadcrumbs, onion, leaves and 1 egg together till smooth. Make the mixture into small sausage-shaped rolls and dip in the beaten egg. Coat with breadcrumbs. Repeat the egg and breadcrumb coating. Deep-fry the rolls four at a time until golden brown. Drain and serve hot.

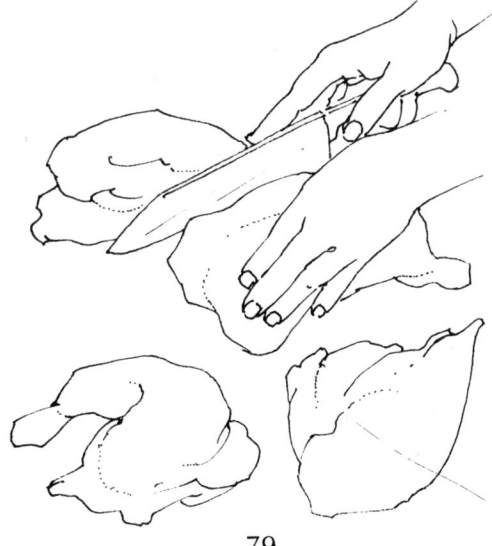

Easy Gougere

This gougere will satisfy any hungry palate.

Ingredients *(Serves 2)*

- 80 g butter
- 1 cup water
- 1 cup plain flour, sifted
- 4 eggs
- 1/2 cup cheese, grated

For Filling
- 50 g butter
- 2 cloves garlic, chopped
- 1/2 cup green shallots, chopped
- 2 tbsp plain flour
- 1 cup of milk
- 1/2 cup water
- 150 g button mushrooms, sliced
- 1/2 cup cheese, grated
- 1 cup chicken, cooked and chopped
- 1 tsp chicken stock powder

Preparation

Bring butter and water to boil in a pan. Keep stirring till the butter is melted. Add the flour all at once and stir well till the mixture leaves the side of the pan. Take the pan off the heat and add eggs one at a time. Beat well with a beater and stir in the cheese. In a large round greased pan, spoon the pastry around and up the sides of the pan leaving a hollow in the centre. Bake in a hot oven till the pastry is browned and puffed. Remove from the oven and fill the hollow with the filling and bake for another 5 minutes.

Filling: Heat the butter and cook the garlic and shallots till soft. Stir in the flour and add the milk gradually. Add the chicken stock powder and water. Heat till the mixture thickens. Stir in the chicken, mushrooms and the cheese. Fill up the pastry with this filling as specified above.

Favourite Quiche

This quiche with its crisp pastry makes a delightful snack for the whole family.

Ingredients *(Serves 2)*

- 1 cup plain flour, sifted with a pinch of salt
- 90 g (3 oz) butter
- 1 egg-yolk, lightly beaten
- 1 tbsp lemon juice

For Filling

- 250 g fish or chicken, cooked and chopped
- 1 cup cream
- 4 rashers bacon, diced and fried in oil till crisp
- 3 eggs
- 1 tbsp grated cheese
- 1 tbsp coriander leaves, chopped
- Salt and pepper to taste

Preparation

Add the butter to the sifted flour and rub till the mixture resembles fine breadcrumbs. Add the egg-yolk and lemon juice and mix to a firm dough . If necessary add 1-2 tsp of water. Knead lightly. Roll out pastry to a circle on a lightly floured surface to fit a round pie dish or flan tin. Fit pastry into the tin gently and with fingers, press into the grooves of the tin. Make sure the pastry does not break. Roll the rolling pin over the top of the tin quickly and firmly to cut off excess pastry. Refrigerate for about an hour. Arrange the chicken or fish in the base of the pastry. Then sprinkle the bacon. Beat together the eggs, cream, leaves, cheese, salt, pepper and pour the egg-mixture over the back of a metal spoon into the pastry. Bake in a moderate oven till the filling has set. This will take about 30 to 40 minutes. Cut into wedges and serve.

Savoury Pie

Pastry making has never been easier. Try this and you'll see why.

Ingredients *(Serves 4)*

- 1 cup plain flour
- 90 g butter
- 1 egg-yolk, lightly beaten
- 1 tbsp lemon juice
- Pinch of salt

For Filling

- 250 g cooked chicken or fish, chopped
- 1 cup cream
- 2 eggs
- 1 tbsp coriander leaves, chopped
- 1 tbsp grated cheese
- Salt and pepper to taste

Preparation

Sift the flour and salt into a bowl. Rub in the butter till it resembles breadcrumbs. Mix to a firm dough with the egg-yolk and lemon juice. If necessary add 1 or 2 tbsp of water. Knead lightly on a lightly floured surface. Roll out the pastry to fit into a 9-inch pie tin. Handle the pastry gently. With fingers, ease the pastry into the tin and press into the grooves of the tin. To make the pastry look neat, roll the rolling pin over the top of the tin quickly and firmly. This will cut off the excess pastry. Refrigerate for 1 hour.

Put the pie tin in an oven tray. Beat the cream, eggs, salt and pepper, coriander leaves, cheese together. Arrange the chicken or fish in base of pastry shell. Pour the egg-mixture over the back of a metal spoon to cover the chicken. Bake in a moderately hot oven for about 10 minutes. Cook a further 1/2 an hour until the filling has set. Serve as a delicious snack as itself or with salad.

Meat Snacks

Beef Crescent Fry

These uncooked crescents can be stored in the freezer and used for those unexpected guests.

Ingredients *(Serves 4)*

- 1 1/2 cups plain sifted flour
- 3/4 cup boiling water
- 1 egg-white, lightly beaten
- Oil for deep-frying

For Filling

- 2 tbsp oil
- 1 onion, chopped
- 2 cloves garlic, chopped
- 1 tsp ginger, chopped
- 2 tsps coriander powder
- 1 tsp chilli powder
- 1/4 kg beef, minced
- 1 teaspoon pepper powder
- Salt to taste
- 2 tsps coriander leaves, chopped

Preparation

In a bowl, add the boiling water to the flour. Knead on a lightly floured surface till smooth. Keep aside for 1/2 an hour. Roll half the dough on a lightly floured surface until 2mm thick. Cut out 8 cm rounds. Put a little of the filling on each round. Brush the edges lightly with the egg-white. Fold rounds in half and press to seal. Just before serving, deep-fry the crescents in hot oil until browned. Drain.

Filling: Heat oil in pan. Add the garlic, ginger and onion. cook for a minute. Add the powders, beef and the rest of the ingredients. Cook till the meat is done. Keep aside to cool.

Hamburgers

There is nothing more safer and healthier than home-made hamburgers. Besides it isn't as difficult as you thought.

Ingredients *(Serves 6)*
- 750 g minced beef
- 1/2 cup bread crumbs
- 1/3 cup milk
- 1 onion, chopped
- 1 tbsp Worcestershire sauce
- 6 hamburger buns
- Salt and pepper to taste

For the Topping
- 1 oz butter or margarine
- 1 onion, sliced into rings
- 1 cup mushrooms, thinly sliced
- 1 tsp Worcestershire sauce

Preparation

Mix the hamburger ingredients. Divide the mixture into 6 and shape into patties. Grill for about 15 minutes till cooked. For the topping, melt the butter in a frying pan. Fry onion till transparent. Add the mushrooms, salt and pepper. Fill each bun with each patty. Top with the onion, mushroom mixture and serve hot.

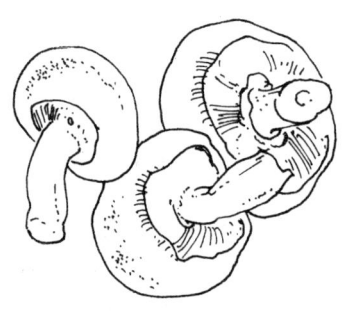

Meatballs and Cheese

For those sudden guests, marinate this mixture and freeze it. At the time of frying, thaw and voila! A snack in no time!

Ingredients *(Serves 4)*

- 400 g beef
- 2 onions, finely chopped
- 1 bunch spring onions, chopped
- 1 tbsp coriander
- 1 tsp soy sauce
- 1 tsp oil
- 1/2 tsp sugar
- 1 tbsp cornflour
- Cheese cubes
- Salt and pepper to taste

Preparation

In a frying pan, fry the coriander until the smell comes and grind it. Set aside. Marinate the meats with the rest of the ingredients except the cheese cubes. Leave it aside for about 1/2 an hour to 45 minutes. Shape the prepared mixture into small balls and deep-fry till golden brown. Cut the cheese cubes into smaller cubes. Secure each meatball on a cheese cube with a toothpick. Serve with cubes of cucumber for the extra crunch.

Meat Tarts

Try these tarts with a simple meat filling. Garnished with mint leaves, these make an absolute delight on the table.

Ingredients *(Serves 3)*

- 1 cup plain flour
- 60 g of butter
- 1 egg-yolk
- 3 teaspoons of lime juice
- Water as needed (about 1 tbsp)

For Filling

- 1 onion, chopped
- 1 teaspoon of ginger ground
- 2 tsps of garlic, ground
- Salt to taste
- 200 g beef, minced
- 1 teaspoon of honey
- 2 tbsp oil

Preparation

Sift the flour into a bowl and rub in the butter till it resembles breadcrumbs. Add the rest of the ingredients to mix to a firm dough. Knead till smooth on a lightly floured surface. Cover and keep in the refrigerator for about 1/2 an hour. Roll pastry out till about 5 mms thick. Cut rounds from the pastry to fit the holes in your tart tin. Prick all over with a fork and bake in a moderate oven till lightly browned. Keep aside to cool. Put a little of the cooked filling into each tart and refrigerate for about 1/2 an hour. Garnish with mint leaves.

Filling: Heat oil in a pan. Add the onions and fry till soft. Add the ginger and garlic till the aroma comes. Add the beef and stir-fry till it loses its colour. Add the honey and salt and stir till cooked. Keep aside to cool.

Bacon Snacks

Horseback Snacks

This is an absolute treat which you must treat yourself to. And yes, your family and friends too. It is exotic!

Ingredients *(Serves 4)*
- 8 large cooked prunes or oysters
- 4 rashers of bacon pepper
- 4 slices thin buttered toast

Preparation
Cook prunes until almost tender and drain well. Stone the prunes. Cut bacon rashers in half and wrap around the prunes. Fasten with cocktail sticks. Grill until bacon is crisp and brown. Serve on toast and dust with pepper. If cooked oysters are used instead of prunes, just season the oysters with salt, pepper and lemon juice to taste. Wrap the bacon rashers around the oysters. Proceed as for the bacon with prunes.

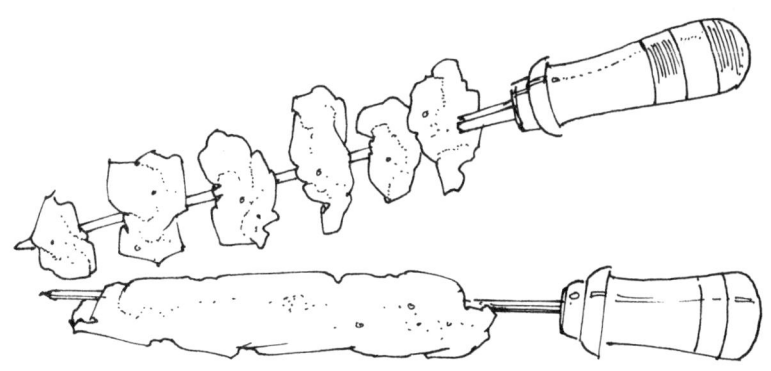

Stuffed Pancakes

Try these stuffed pancakes for a fantastic snack. Let your imagination run wild and fill the pancakes up with your favourite filling.

Ingredients *(Serves 4-6)*

- 4 oz flour
- Pinch of salt
- 1 egg
- 280 ml milk or equal quantity of milk and water

For Filling

- 4 oz bacon
- 1 small onion, chopped
- 1/2 cup mushrooms (sliced)
- 2 or 3 tomatoes, chopped
- Salt and pepper
- Cheese or tomato sauce

Preparation

Sift the flour and salt. Add the egg and enough milk or milk and water to give a creamy consistency. Beat well.

Remove rinds from the bacon. Fry the rinds to get fat. In the same fat, fry the onion, chopped bacon, mushrooms, tomatoes, salt and pepper to taste. Make the pancakes and spread each of them with the filling. Roll the pancakes with the filling inside or line the pancakes one on top of the other with the filling spread in between. Top with grated cheese and grill in a hot oven for 5 minutes. Garnish with parsley and tomato slices.

Instant Savoury Pie

The tiny cubes of bread on top make this dish serve as a garnish as well as an accompaniment.

Ingredients *(Serves 6)*

- 500 kg minced meat
- cup uncooked rice
- 1 cup tomato puree
- 1 onion, chopped
- Salt and pepper to taste
- 40 g butter
- 4 slices of bread, buttered and cut into cubes.

Preparation

Fry the onion in the butter. Add the rest of the ingredients except the bread cubes. Mix well and bring it to the boil. Simmer for about 1/2 an hour and spread the mixture in a flat greased dish. Sprinkle the prepared bread on top and bake for 15 minutes at 325° F/160° C. Grill for a further 5 minutes till the top is crisp.

Quick and Easy Pizza

This is probably the easiest pizza you can make.

Ingredients *(Serves 4)*

- 4 hamburger buns
- 60 g butter, melted
- 16 slices of salami or ham
- Cheese slices
- Tomato sauce
- Pepper to taste

Preparation

Cut the buns in half and spread the butter on each half. Toast lightly and spread with tomato sauce. Top with the salami or ham and put the cheese slices on top. Sprinkle the pepper and put it back under the grill till the cheese is melted. Serve hot.

Minced Meat Loaf

This is not your regular bread loaf but a meat loaf.

Ingredients *(Serves 8)*

- 1 kg minced meat
- 1 cup tomato puree
- 1 egg
- 2 tbsp tomato sauce
- Salt and pepper to taste
- 1 tbsp chicken stock powder

Preparation

Preheat the oven. Put the mince in a large bowl and mix with the rest of the ingredients, excluding the tomato sauce. Stir till well mixed and shape firmly into a loaf. Place in a greased loaf pan. Bake for an hour. Check if there is any fat. Gently tip the pan and remove the fat. Spread the tomato sauce on top of the loaf and return to the oven. Bake for another 1/2 an hour and serve either hot or cold.

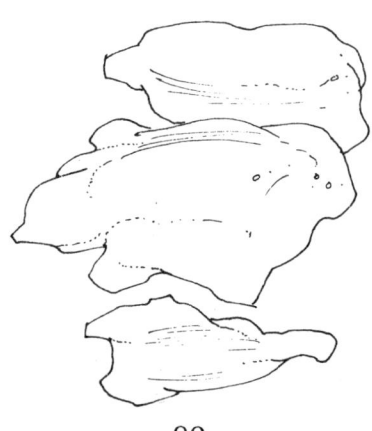

Fried Meat Cakes

The fried onions added into this snack gives an extra flavour which is hard to resist.

Ingredients *(Serves 4)*
- 3 potatoes, boiled and mashed
- 2 tsp butter
- 1 onion, sliced and fried in hot oil till light brown
- 75 g minced mutton or beef, fried
- 1 egg, beaten
- 2 tbsp plain flour
- Oil for deep-frying

Preparation

In a bowl, mix the fried onion with the fried meat, butter, salt and pepper. Add the mashed potatoes and mix well. Shape into balls which are slightly flattened. Dip in the flour and then in the beaten egg. Deep-fry till golden brown and drain on kitchen paper. Serve hot in a plate garnished with tomatoes, cucumber, lettuce and mint leaves. Don't forget the tomato sauce.

TIPS

- Put a spoonful of dry rice in your biscuit tin and the biscuits will not lose their crispness.
- When cooking pulao, add the juice of 1 lemon into the pot. Rice grains will be white and separate.
- When chewing gum is stuck to clothes, rub a piece of ice and it will come off.
- To sharpen a pair of blunt scissors, cut a few pieces of sandpaper and it will be sharp again.
- To save energy and water, first clean greasy pots and pans with old newspaper crumbled into balls. Then wash off with hot water.
- Salt sprinkled into a frying pan will prevent food from sticking to the bottom of the pan and also keep oil from splashing.
- If your cutlets cannot be shaped properly, soak some bread in water for a few minutes and drain well. Add to the cutlet mixture and proceed to make cutlets. If there are no breadcrumbs when you need to make cutlets, no need to fret, use semolina (rava) instead.
- If your sugar has become moist due to humidity, spread on a clean cloth in hot sun for about 1-2 hours and it will become dry again.
- To prevent your eyes from watering when cutting onions, place whole unpeeled onions in a bowl of water and then peel.

GLOSSARY

FOODGRAINS

English	Spiked millet	Barley	Jowar	Italian millet	Maize (dry)	Oatmeal	Ragi
Hindi	Bajra	Jau	Juar-janera	Kangri	Makai	Jai	Okra
Tamil	Cambu	Barli arisi	Cholam	Thenai	Muka cholam	—	Ragi
Telugu	Gantelu	Barli biyyam	Jonnalu	Korralu	Mekka jonnalu	—	Chollu
Marathi	Bajri	Juv	Jwari	Rala	Muka	Jai	Nachni
Bengali	Bajra	Job	Juar	Syamadhan kangni	Sukna paka bhutta	—	—
Gujarati	Bajri	Jau	Juar	Ral kang	Makai	—	Ragi bhav
Malayalam	Kamboo	Yavam	Cholam	Thina	Unakku cholam	Oat mavu	Moothari (korra)
Kannada	—	—	Jola	—	Vonugida musikinu	Jolu	Ragi
Kashmiri	Ping	Wushku	—	Shol	Makka'y	Khaj	—

Contd...

Foodstuff	Rice (raw)	Rice (parboiled)	Rice (white)	Rice (black)	Rice flakes	Rice (puffed)	Samai
Hindi	Arwa chawal	Usna chawal	Safed chaval	Chaval (kala)	Chowla	Murmura	Kutki, Sanwali
Tamil	Pachai arisi	Puzhungal arisi	Vellai puttu arisi	Karuppu puttu arisi	Arisi aval	Arisia pori	Samai
Telugu	Pachi biyyam	Uppudu biyyam	Thella biyyam	Nalla biyyam	Atukulu	Murmuralu	—
Marathi	Tandool	Tandool ukda	—	—	Pohe	Murmure	Sava
Bengali	Atap chowl	Siddha chowl	—	—	Chaler khood	Muri	Kangni
Gujarati	Hatna	Ukadelloo chokha	—	—	Pohva	Mumra	—
Malayalam	Pacchari	Puzhungal ari	Velutha puttari	Karutha puttari	Avil	Pori	Puri
Kannada	Kotnuda	Kotnuda	—	—	Avalukki	—	Sur
Kashmiri	Tomul	Behul tomul	—	—	Chidwa	Tolmud bhat	—

Contd...

English	Semolina	Vermicelli	Wheat (whole)	Wheat flour (whole)	Wheat flour (refined)	Wheat (broken)
Hindi	Sooji	Siwain	Gehun	Atta	Maida	Daliya
Tamil	Ravai	Semiya	Godumai	Muzhu godmai ma	Maida mavu	Godhumbi ravai
Telugu	Rawa	Semiya	Godhumalu	Godhum pindi	Maidha pindi	Dinchina gadhumalu
Marathi	—	Shevaya	Gahu	Gahu kuneek	Gahu kuneek	Gavache satva
Bengali	Suji	Sewai	Gomasta	Atta	Maida	Bhanga gom
Gujarati	—	—	Ghau	Ato	—	Fadia ghaun
Malayalam	Rava	Semiya	Muzhu gothambu	Gothambu mavu	Maidu tha gothambu mavu	Gothumbu ari
Kannada	—	Shavige	Godhi	Godhi	Hittu madia	Kuttida Godhi
Kashmiri	Sooj	Ku' nu'	Kanak	Oat	Med	—

VEGETABLES

English	Ash gourd	Bitter gourd	Bottle gourd	Brinjal	Broad beans	Cabbage	Capsicum
Hindi	Safed petha	Karela	Ghia	Baingan	Sem	Bandhgobi	Simla mirch
Bengali	Chal kumdo	karala	Laoo	Begoon	Sheem	Badha kopee	Lonka
Assamese	Lao bishesh	—	Jati lao	Bengena	Urahi	Bondhakobi	Kashmiri jalakai
Oriya	Pani kakkaru	—	Lau	Baigana	Shimba	Patrokobi	Simla lonka
Marathi	Kohala	Karle	Dudhi	Wangi	Ghewda	Pan kobi	Bhopli mirchi
Gujarati	Petha	Karela	Dudhi	Ringna	Papdi	Kobi	Simla marchan
Telugu	Boodie gumadi	Kakara	Sorakaya	Vankaya	Pedda chikkudu	Kosu	Pedda mirappa
Kannada	Budu gumbala	Hagalkai	Sorekai	Badanekai	Chapparadavare	Kosu	Donne menasinakai
Tamil	Pooshanikkai	Pavakkai	Suraikai	Kaththarikai	Avaraikai	Muttaikosu	Kuda milakai
Malayalam	Kumbalanga	Kaypakka	Cheraikai	Vazhutheninga	Amarakai	Muttakose	Parangi mulagu
Kashmiri	Masha'ly al	Karelu	Poerimal	Waangun	—	Bandgobhi	Simla Mirch

Contd...

English	Carrot	Cauliflower	Cluster beans	Colocasia	Coriander leaves	Cucumber	Curry leaves
Hindi	Gajar	Phulgobi	Guar ki phalli	Arvi	Hara Dhania	Khira	Kadi patta
Bengali	Gajar	Foolcopy	Jhar sim	—	Dhonay pata	Sasha	Curry pata
Assamese	Gajor	Phoolkobi	—	Kochu	Dhania paat	—	Narasingha paat
Oriya	Gajar	Phulakobi	—	—	Dhania patra	—	Bhrusanga patta
Marathi	Gajar	Fulkobi	Govari	Alu kanda	Kothimbir	Kakari	Kadhi patta
Gujarati	Gajar	Fool kobi	Govar	Alvi	Kothmir	Kakdi	Mitho limdo
Telugu	Gajjara	Cauliflower	Goruchikkudu kayalu	Chamadumpa	Kothimeera	Dosakaya	Kariveppaku
Kannada	Gajjari	Hookosu	Gorikayi	Keshave	Kottambari soppu	Southaikayi	Karibevu
Tamil	Carrot	Koveppu	Kothavarangai	Seppann kizhangu	Koththamali ilaigal	Kakkarikkai	Kariveppilai
Malayalam	Carrot	Coliflower	Kothavara	Chembu	Kothamalli ila	Vellari	Kariveppila
Kashmiri	Gazar	Phoolgobhi	—	—	Daniwal	Laa'r	—

Contd...

English	Drumstick	French beans	Garlic	Ginger (fresh)	Green chillies	Jackfruit	Lady's finger
Hindi	Sahjan ki phali	Pharsbeen	Lassan	Adrak	Hari mirch	Kathal	Bhindi
Bengali	Sajane dauta	French beans	Rasoon	Ada (tatka)	Kancha lonka	Echore	Dhanroce
Assamese	Sajina	Faras been	Naharoo	Ada (kesa)	Kesa jalakia	—	Bhendi
Oriya	Sajana chhuin	French beans	Rasuna	Ada (kancha)	Kancha lonka	—	Bhendi
Marathi	Shevgyachya shenga	Farasbi	Lasun	Aale	Hirvya mirchya	Kawla phanas	Bhendi
Gujarati	Saragvani shing	Fansi	Lasan	Adu	Lila marcha	Phunas	Bhinda
Telugu	Munagakayalu	French chikkudu	Vellulli	Allam (pachchi)	Pachchi mirapakayalu	Letha panasa	Bendakaaya
Kannada	Nuggekai	Avare	Bellulli	Ashi Shunti	Hasi menasinakai	Yele halasu	Bendekai
Tamil	Murungaikai	Beans	Ulli Poondu	Inji	Pachchai milagai	Pila pinchu	Vendaikai
Malayalam	Muringakkaya	Beans	Veluthulli	Inji	Pachamulagu	Idichakka	Vendakka
Kashmiri	—	—	Ruhan	Adrak	Nyool martsu waungun	—	Bindu

Contd...

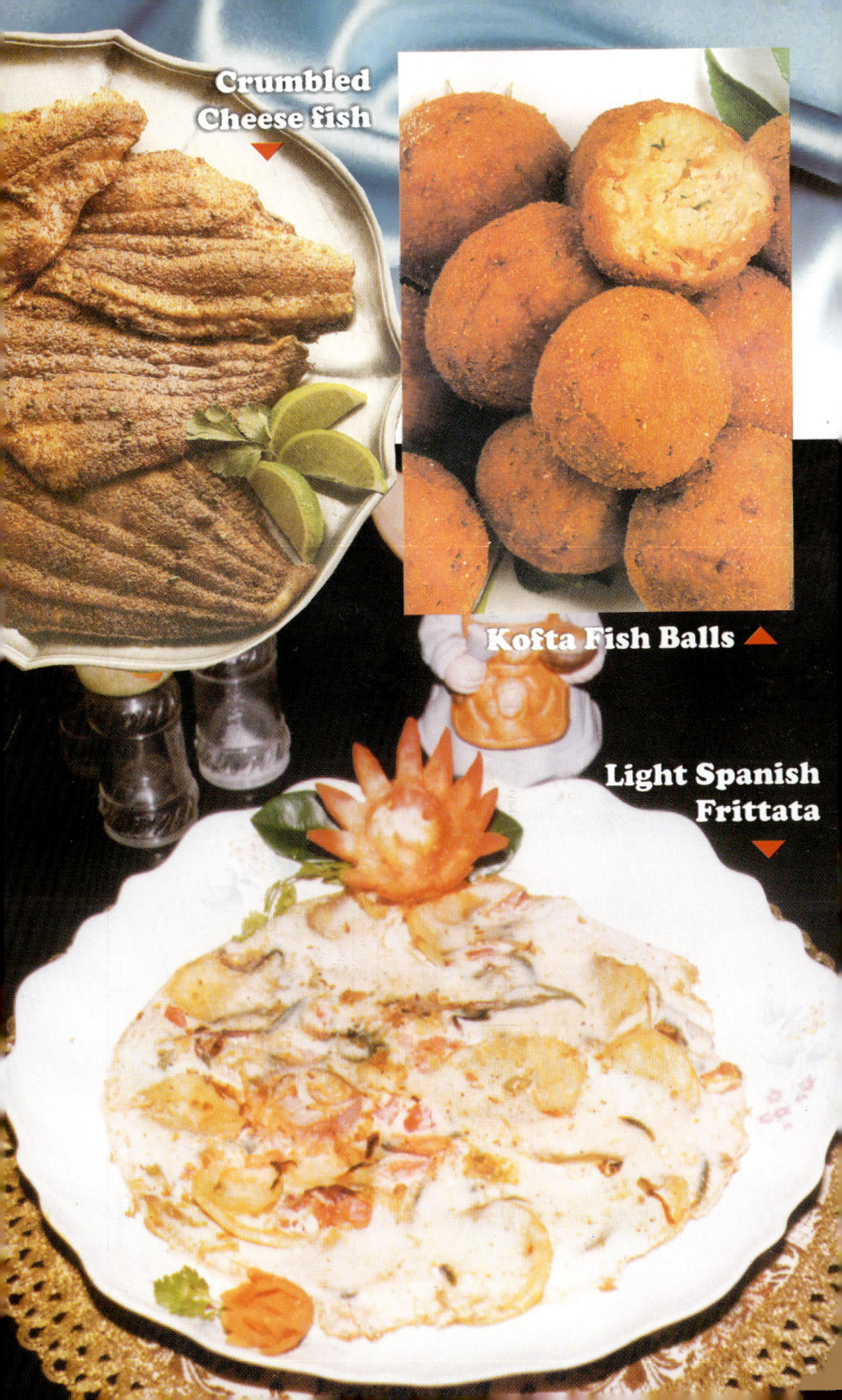

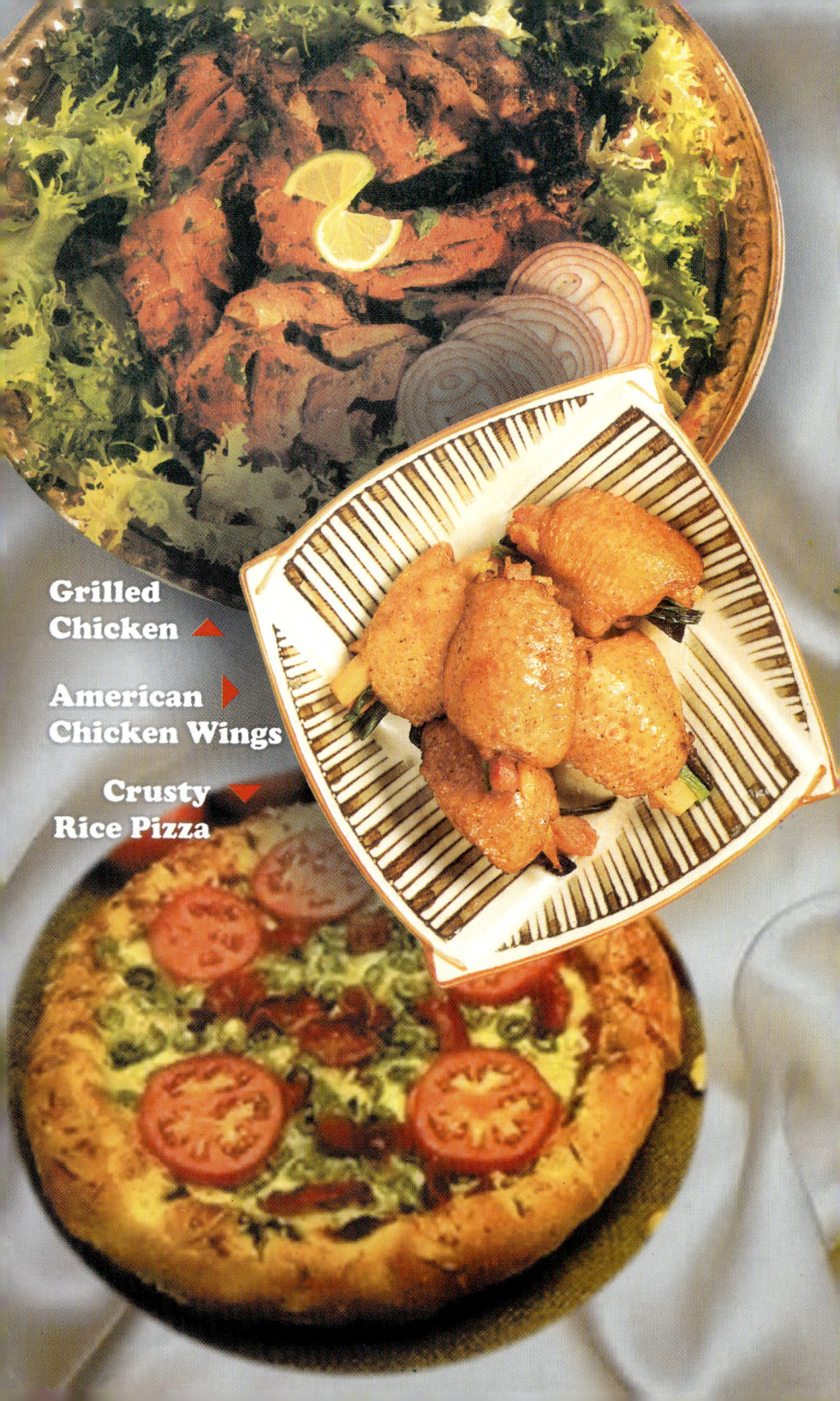
- Grilled Chicken
- American Chicken Wings
- Crusty Rice Pizza

English	Lettuce	Lemon	Mint leaves	Onion	Parwal	Peas	Plantain flower	Plantain green
Hindi	Salad ke patte	Nimbu	Pudina	Pyaz	Parwal	Matar	kele ka phool	Kacha kela
Bengali	Lettuce	Lebu	Poodina pata	Pyaz	Potol	Motor	Mocha	Kancha kala
Assamese	Laipaat	Nemu	Podina	—	Patol	Motormah	—	—
Oriya	Lettuce	Lembu	Podana patra	—	Potala	Matar	Kel phool	Kele
Marathi	Saladchi paane	Limbu	Pudina	Kanda	—	Matar	Kelphool	Kela
Gujarati	Lettuce	Limbu	Fudino	Dungli	—	Vatana	Aratipuwu	Arati kayi
Telugu	Lettuce koora	Nimma	Pudhina koora	Nirulli	—	Bathanedu	Balo mothu	Bala kayi
Kannada	Lettuce soppu	Nimbu	Pudina sopu	Erulli	—	Betani	Vazhaippu	Vazhaikkai
Tamil	Lettuce keerai	Elumicham pazham	Pudhinaa	Vengayam	—	Pattani	Vazhappoo	Vazhakka
Malayalam	Uvarcheera	Cherunaranga	Pudhinaa	Ulli	—	Pattani Payaru	—	—
Kashmiri	Salaad	Num	Pudine	Gandu	—	Matar	—	—

Contd...

English	Plantain stem	Potato	Radish	Red pumpkin	Ridge gourd	Snake gourd	Sweet potato	Yam elephant
Hindi	Kele ka tana	Aloo	Muli	Sitaphal	Torai	Chichinga	Shakarkand	Zaminkand
Bengali	Thor	Aloo	Mulo	Ronga Koomra	Jhinge	—	Rangalu	Kham aloo
Assamese	—	Alu	—	Ronga lao	—	—	—	Kaath aloo
Oriya	—	Alu	—	Kakharu	—	—	—	Deshi alu
Marathi	Kelecha khunt	Batate	Mula	Lal bhopla	Dodka	Pudwal	Ratale	Suran
Gujarati	Kelanu thed	Batata	Mula	Kolu	Turai	Pandola	Sakkaria	Suran
Telugu	Arati davva	Bangaala dumpa	Mullangi	Erra gummadi	Beerakai	Potlakayi	Dumpalu	Kanda dumpa
Kannada	Dindu	Aalugadde	Mullangi	Kempu kumbala	Heeraikai	Padavalai	Genasu	Suvarnagadde
Tamil	Vazhaithandu	Urulaikizhangu	Mullangi	Parangikai	Pirrkkankai	Podalangai	Sarkarai valli kizhangu	Chenai kizhangu
Malayalam	Vazhappindi	Uralakkizhangu	Mullangi	Chuvappu mathan	Pecchinga	Padavalanga	Chakkara kizhangu	Chena
Kashmiri	—	Oloo	Muj	Paarimal	Turrelu	—	—	—

PULSES

English	Bengal gram (whole)	Bengal gram (split)	Black gram (split)	Black gram (whole)	Cornflour	Cow gram	Green gram (whole)
Hindi	Chana	Chana dal	Urad dal	Sabat urad	Makai ka atta	Lobia (bada)	Moong
Bengali	Chola	Banglar chhola	Mashkolair dal	Mashkolai dal	Bhoottar maida	Barbati	Mug
Assamese	—	Buttor dail	Matir dail (phola)	Matir dail (gota)	Moida	—	—
Oriya	—	Buta (chhota)	Biri (phala)	Biri (gota)	Makka atta	—	—
Marathi	Hurbhura	Chana dal	Udid dal	Udid	Makyache pith	Kuleeth	Mug
Gujarati	Chana	Chana nidaal	Adad ni dal	Adad	Makai no lot	—	Mag
Telugu	Sanagalu	Senaga pappu	Mina pappu	Minu mulu	Mokkajonnalu (pindi)	Ada chandalu	Pesalu
Kannada	Kadale	Kadale bela	Uddina bela	Uddu	Musukinajolada hittu	Thadaguni	Hesaru kalu
Tamil	Muzhu kadalai	Kadalai paruppu	Ulutham paruppu	Ulundhu	Chola Maavu	Karamani	Pachai payaru
Malayalam	Kadala	Kadala parippu	Uzhunnu parrippu	Uzhunnu	Cholapodi	Payar	Cherupayaru
Kashmiri	Chanu	Chanu dal	Maha dal	Maha	Makai Oat	Mooth	Muang

Contd...

English	Green gram (split)	Horse gram	Kesari dal	Kidney beans	Red gram	Red lentils	Soya bean
Hindi	Moong dal	Kulthi	Lang dal	Rajma	Arhar dal	Masoor dal	Bhat
Bengali	Moog	Kulthi kalai	Khesari	Barbati beej	Arhar dal	Lal masoor (bhanga)	Gari kalai
Assamese	Sevjiy Boot	—	—	Markhowa urahi	Rahor dail	Masoor dail (phola)	—
Oriya	Muga (Phala)	—	—	Baragudi chhuin	Harada dali	Masura dali (phala)	—
Marathi	Moog dal	Kuleeth	Lakh dal	—	Tur dal	Masur dal	Soya
Gujarati	Magnidal	Kuleeth	Lakh	—	Tuver dal	Masur dal	Soya
Telugu	Pesaru pappu	Ulavalu	Lamka pappu	—	Kandi pappu	Missu pappu	—
Kannada	Hesare bele	Huruli	—	—	Togar bele	Masur bele	—
Tamil	Pasi paruppu	Kollu	Vattuparuppu	—	Thuvaram parappu	Massor paruppu	—
Malayalam	Cherupayar parippu	Muthira	—	—	Thuvara parippu	Masoor parippu	Soya bean
Kashmiri	Muang dal	Gur chana	—	Rajma	Arhar	Musur	Soya

FRUITS AND DRY FRUITS

English	Almond	Coconut	Currants	Dates	Dry plums
Hindi	Badam	Nariyal	Mungaqqa	Khajur	Alu bukhara
Bengali	Badam	Narcole	Manaca	Khejoor	Sookno kool
Assamese	Badam	Narikol	Kismis	Khejur	Sukan bogori
Oriya	Badaam	Nadia	Kala kismis	Khajura	Barakoli jateeya phala
Marathi	Badam	Naral	Manuka	Khajur	Alubhukar
Gujarati	Badam	Naliyer	Kalli draksh	Khajoor	Suka Plum
Telugu	Badam	Kobbari kaaya	Endu nalla dhraksha	Kharjoora pandu	—
Kannada	Badami	Tenginakai	Dweepa dharakshi-kappu	Kharjoora	—
Tamil	Badam/vadhumai	Thengai	Karumdhraakshai	Perichampazham	Aalpacota ular pazham
Malayalam	Badam	Nalikeram/Thenga	Karuthamurthiri	Eethapazham	—
Kashmiri	Badam	Narjil	Kismish	Khazur	Sok Ear

Contd...

English	Guavas	Lemon	Orange	Raisins	Walnuts
Hindi	Amrud	Nimbu	Santra	Kishmish	Akhrot
Bengali	Payara	Lebu	Kamla lebu	Kishmish	Akhrot
Assamese	Madhurium	Nemu	Sumothira	Sukan angoor	Akhrot
Oriya	Pijuli	Lembu	Kamala	Kismis	Akhrot
Marathi	Peru	Limbu	Santre	Bedane	Akrod
Gujarati	Jamrukh	Limbu	Santara	Lal draksh	Akhrot
Telugu	Jaamapandu	Nimma	Kamala Pandu	Kismis pallu	Aakrot
Kannada	Seebe	Nimbe	Kittale	Dweepadrakshi	Acrota
Tamil	Koyyapazham	Elumicham pazham	Kichilipazham	Ular dhraakshai	Akhrot
Malayalam	Perakkai	Cherunaranga	Madhura naranga	Unakkamunthiri	Akrotandi
Kashmiri	—	Neum	Santar	Kishmish	Dun

DRY SPICES

English	Aniseed	Asafoetida	Basil leaves	Bay leaf	Caraway seeds	Cardamom (brown)	Cardamom (green)	Cinnamon
Hindi	Saunf	Hing	Tulse ke patte	Tej patta	Shahjeera	Moti elaichi	Choti elaichi	Dalchini
Bengali	Mowri	Hing	Tulsi pata	Tej pata	Sajeera	Elach (tamate)	Elach (sobooj)	Daroochini
Assamese	Guwamari	Hing	Tulosi paat	Tejpaat	Bilati jira	Ilachi (muga)	Ilachi (sevjia)	Dalcheni
Oriya	Panamahuri	Hengu	Tulasi patra	Teja patra	Sahajira	Aleicha	Gijuratie	Dalachini
Marathi	Badishep	Hing	Tulsichi pancy	Tamal patra	Shahjeera	Masala welchi	Welchi (hirvi)	Dalchini
Gujarati	Varyali	Hing	Tulsina pan	Tamal patra	Jiru	Elcho	Lila alchi	Tuj
Telugu	Sopaginja	Inguva	Thulasi akulu	—	Seema sopyginjale	Yalakulu	Yala kulu (pachavi)	Dalchina chekka
Kannada	Sopubeeja	Hingu	Tulasi ele	—	Caraway beejagalre	Yalakki	Yalakki (hasuru)	Dalchini
Tamil	Perumjeerakam	Perungaayam	Thulasi	—	Karunjeerakam	Elakkai (Pazhuppu)	Elakkai (pachchai)	Lavangapattai
Malayalam	Perumjeerakam	Kaayam	Tulasi	—	Karunjeerakam	Elakkaya	Pach Elakkaya	Karuvapatta
Kashmiri	Badyaan	Yangu	—	Jalwathar/Krhun Zur	—	—	Aal	Dalchin

Contd...

English	Cloves	Coriander seeds	Cumin seeds	Fenugreek seeds	Mace	Mustard seeds	Nutmeg	Parsley
Hindi	Laung	Sukha dhania	Jeera	Methi dana	Javitri	Rai	Jaiphal	Ajmooda ka patta
Bengali	Labango	Dhonay	Jeera	Methi	Jacetri	Sarsay	Jaifall	Parsley
Assamese	Long	Dhania guti	Gota jeera	Paleng	Jance	Sarioh guti	Jaaiphal	Sugandhi lota
Oriya	Labanga	Dhania	Jira	Methi	Jayatree	Sorisha	Jaiphala	Balabalua shaga
Marathi	Lavanga	Dhane	Jire	Methi dane	Jaypatri	Mohari	Jayphal	Ajmoda
Gujarati	Laving	Dhana	Jeeru	Methi	Jaypatra	Rai	Jaypal	Ajmo
Telugu	Lavangalu	Dhaniyalu	Jeelakara	Menthulu	Japathri	Aavaalu	Jaikaaya	Kothimeerajati koora
Kannada	Lavanga	Kottambari beeja	Jeerige	Menthe	Japatri	Sasive kalu	Jaike	Kottambari jotiya soppu
Tamil	Kraambu	Kaththamali virai	Jeerakam	Vendhayam	Jaadipathri	Kadugu	Jaadhikai	Kothamallu ilaigal pole
Malayalam	Karayaamboovu	Kathamalli	Jeerakam	Uluva	Jathipathri	Kadugu	Jathikka	Malliela pole
Kashmiri	Ru'ang	Daaniwal	Zyur	Meth Bual	Jawitri	Asur	Zaiphal	

Contd...

100

English	Peppercorns	Pomegranate seeds	Poppy seeds	Red Chillies	Tamarind	Turmeric	Vinegar	Thymol
Hindi	Kali mirch ke daane	Anardana	Khus khus	Lal mirch	Imli	Haldi	Sirka	Ajwain
Bengali	Marich	Dareem bij	Posto	Paka lonka	Tentool	Halood	Seerka	—
Assamese	Jaluk	Dalim guti	—	Sukan jalakia	Teteli	Halodhi	Sirika	—
Oriya	Golamaricha	Dalimba manji	—	Nali lankamaricha	Tentuli	Haladi	Vinegar	Onva
Marathi	Kale Miri	Dalimbache dane	Khas khas	Lal mirchya	Chincha	Halad	Sirka	Ajmo
Gujarati	Mari	Dadamna bee	Khaskhas	Lal marcha	Amli	Haldar	Sirko	—
Telugu	Miriyaalu	Daanimma ginjalu	Gasagasaalu	Erra mirapa kayalu	Chinthapandu	Pasupu	—	—
Kannada	Menasina kalu	Dalimbo beeja	Gasagase beeja	Kempu menasinakai	Hunase hannu	Arasina	—	—
Tamil	Milagu	Maadhulai vidhai	Kasakasaa	Milagai vatal	Puli	Manjal	Pulikaadi	—
Malayalam	Kurumulagu	Madhala naranga kuru-	—	Chuvanna Mulagu	Puli	Manjal	Vinagiri	—
Kashmiri	Kruhun March	Anar dan	Kashkash	Wazul march waongun	Tombar	Ledar	Sirk	Jaoand

ACKNOWLEDGEMENTS

My appreciation to my husband, Dr Mathew Abraham for always encouraging and pushing me forward. Thank you for all those late nights you stayed up for me. I cannot thank you enough.

Thanks to my children, Satshya, Prethyash and Sneha for giving me the time and space to write. Thank you for being who you are.

Thanks to my parents, Dr & Mrs John Jacob for setting the precedent of writing books and giving me all the encouragement I ever needed to make my dreams a reality.

Thanks to Dr & Mrs Kurien Abraham, Mr & Mrs Jacob Cheriyan, Dr. Kurien P. Abraham, Mr & Mrs John Thomas and Dr Blessy Abraham for everything.

Thanks to Ammu, Annu, Beena, Maria, Razia, Valsa and Zarina who make each Thursday a special day.

Thank to Maria Abraham, for making sure she reads my articles.

Thank you, Corrine Dempsey for telling me to keep writing.

Thank you to all my close family friends in Singapore who have been a precious part of my good memories. You have encouraged me tremendously.

Above all, thanks to my Saviour Jesus Christ, without whom none of this would have been possible.

—Elizabeth Jyothi Mathew

Books on Cookery

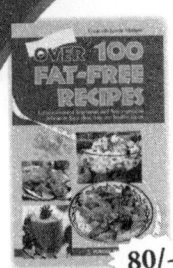
80/-

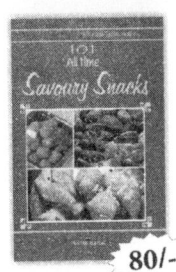
80/-

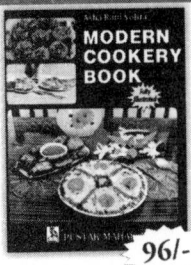
96/-

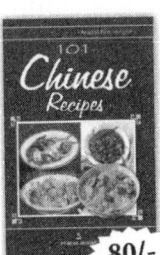
80/-

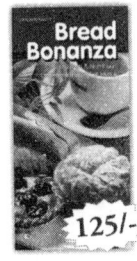
125/-
In Colour

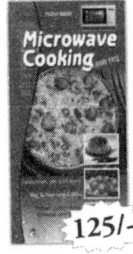
125/-
In Colour

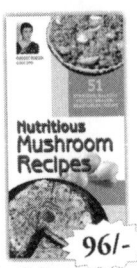
96/-
In Colour

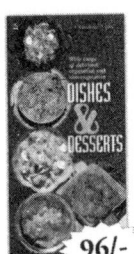
96/-

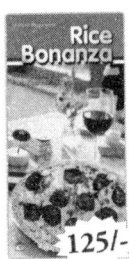
125/-
In Colour

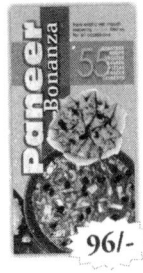
96/-

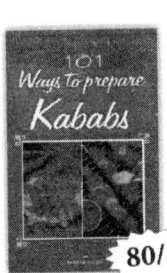
80/-

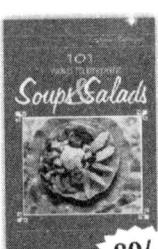
80/-

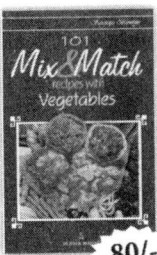
80/-

Postage: Extra